SIX MONTHS TO CHANGE THE WORLD

Pierre Dukan

SIX MONTHS TO CHANGE THE WORLD

Learn the importance of eating right during
the last six months of your pregnancy to
protect your child's health

JOHN BLAKE

Published by John Blake Publishing Ltd,
3 Bramber Court, 2 Bramber Road,
London W14 9PB, England

www.johnblakebooks.com

www.facebook.com/johnblakebooks 🖪
twitter.com/jblakebooks 🖪

ISBN: 978 1 78606 450 9

British Library Cataloguing-in-Publication Data:

A catalogue record for this book is available from the British Library.

Design by www.envydesign.co.uk

Printed in Great Britain by CPI Group (UK) Ltd

1 3 5 7 9 10 8 6 4 2

The information provided in this book is designed to provide helpful information on the
subjects discussed. This book is not meant to be used, nor should it be used, to diagnose or
treat any medical condition. For diagnosis or treatment of any medical problem, consult your
own physician. The publisher and author are not responsible for any specific health or allergy
needs that may require medical supervision and are not liable for any damages or negative
consequences from any treatment, action, application or preparation, to any person reading
or following the information in this book. References are provided for informational
purposes only and do not constitute endorsement of any websites or other sources.
Readers should be aware that the websites listed in this book may change.

Papers used by John Blake Publishing are natural, recyclable products made from
wood grown in sustainable forests. The manufacturing processes conform to the
environmental regulations of the country of origin.

Every attempt has been made to contact the relevant copyright-holders, but some were
unobtainable. We would be grateful if the appropriate people could contact us.

John Blake Publishing is an imprint of Bonnier Publishing
www.bonnierpublishing.co.uk

I dedicate this book to the women in my life:
my mother, my wife and my daughter, but also all the
women of the world who ardently desire the best for
the child they bring into the world.

Contents

Introduction

I've worked on many projects in my life, but the one I'm presenting to you here is without a doubt the most exciting, meaningful and consequential, for me and for my readers alike.

It is my deepest hope that the plan found in this book will help stop the spread of an epidemic that causes immense amounts of suffering. This hope is the motivation for every page and every word.

CHANGING THE WORLD. It's a bold objective, intended to create a stir. It's meant to draw attention to a fact that is all too often covered up or ignored. Humanity today – those now living and the generations that will follow us – faces a grave threat. Statistics from around the world show that this danger has been in our midst for two generations now. In the post-war year, overweight persons numbered in the hundreds of millions; since then, the number has skyrocketed to 2 billion. The problem has a wider reach than ever before.

The crisis of excess weight, obesity and diabetes has long been treated as a somewhat trivial issue. This has been due sometimes to short-sightedness, and sometimes to complicity. But we now know that weight problems are a true scourge. They pollute, impair and otherwise affect the life and well-being of one out of two adults in the West, directly or indirectly leading to the death of 75 million people.[1]

Changing the entire world is the goal, because almost no country has been able to stop the scourge.

SIX MONTHS: Does this mean that the world will be vastly different just six months after the plan is published? No. What it means is that:

- if every pregnant woman understands the idea that what she eats during her pregnancy can radically change the life of her child, and makes decisions accordingly;
- if she understands and accepts that many of the foods she's now consuming are tolerable for her but may not be tolerated by her unborn child; and
- if the plan laid out in this book reaches these women, is properly understood and appeals to their common sense and their keen maternal instincts,

---

[1] Source: World Health Organization (WHO), 'Obesity and Diabetes', Fact Sheet #311, Epidemiological Survey, 2009 (All notes are from the author).

then I believe the plan could truly change the world in terms of the coming generation – the one that will follow the two generations that have borne this scourge.

SIX MONTHS: This refers to the final six months of pregnancy, particularly the fourth and fifth months – sixty crucial days – when the baby's pancreas develops and begins secreting insulin.

SIX MONTHS in which it's well worth considering that the process for manufacturing a human infant was developed at a time when there were no:

- bakeries
- refined sugar
- white flour
- fizzy drinks
- mass-produced breads
- corn flakes
- other industrially processed foods.

Nor was our massive selection of snack foods available – not millions of years ago, nor when your grandmother was carrying your mother in her womb.

SIX MONTHS: A period during which a mother, origin of human life, prepares to give birth. A time when, influenced by maternal hormones, sensing instinctively what might pose a risk to her baby, she is capable of choosing to change her status from 'consumer' to 'mother'.

When I recommended to one of my patients, who was

at the start of her pregnancy, that she follow this plan, she responded with a wonderful crystallisation of my thought. 'Basically,' she said, 'you're asking me to eat for six months the way people ate in my grandmother's time.'

CHAPTER 1

Introducing the Project

The project that is the subject of this book developed slowly, and took shape later than I would have liked. Most of my energy during that period was taken up by a daily frontal attack on my patients' problems with excess weight, obesity and diabetes.

Early on, I started moving away from the dogma that focused on calories. At the end of my ten years of medical studies, I became extremely frustrated as I discovered that what I had been taught was proving very ineffective.

I quickly formed a suspicion, one that never left me: that the calorie theory was based on an unfounded assumption; that not all calories were equal; and that what really mattered was the *type* of calorie, or the nutrient it carried.

In talking with my patients, I found that the vast majority gained weight from eating too many 'invasive carbohydrates' (those that move with ease and enter the blood rapidly and at once).

Over time, I built a method, step by step, that eliminated these 'sugars' during a relatively brief period of weight loss. The results of this method confirmed that excess weight was a condition that could be mastered by those who had the motivation to give up these 'sugars' during the weight-loss phase.

I went on to share this method in books that were widely read, reaching readers all over the world.

Reaching millions of readers is quite a success, but a reader is not a patient. Nonetheless, if a reader has a powerful desire that comes from deep within – if they have what I call DLW, Determination to Lose Weight – that reader, book in hand, will succeed in shedding pounds, and often in maintaining their new weight.

But there are many whose motivation hasn't reached this level, who don't have a strong relationship with a doctor and who suffer from a wealth of misinformation. In the fight against excess weight, these individuals are simply outmatched.

Why is it so hard for them? There are two main reasons.

First, because people who gain weight do so because, despite their aversion to the extra pounds, they can't resist foods that make them fat. This is partly because lobbies for the industry built around sugar, white flour and foods based on these products – in conjunction with the pharmaceutical industry – are violently opposed to anything that could in any way threaten their prosperity.

From birth to the age of fifty, we are bombarded with pressure to eat industrially processed foods that cause us to gain weight. Then, from the age of fifty on, we try to protect our health with extremely expensive drugs for weight-related diseases. It's hard for regular people to grasp the enormous power of the major food producers, or the extent of their ties to the medical community and the media.

So are those who suffer from excess weight a lost cause? Absolutely not. I know from long experience that excess weight, obesity and even diabetes are treatable, even reversible. But success depends on the patient accepting the only effective treatment there is: diet. Any solutions that reject or ignore diet, offering 'nutritional balancing' or just 'listening to your feelings' instead, are illusions: they inspire wonderful dreams, but they lead nowhere.

To combat this powerlessness, I've tried to avoid the usual obstacles and instead taken another path. In doing so, I've constructed – step by step, one element at a time – the complete plan you'll find in this book.

How it all began

I came into the world around the same time as the obesity crisis. I was beginning my medical studies in a period when, to the dismay of health and medical institutions, the number of overweight people in France had reached 1 million. Later – even as I practised nutrition with patients who showed on a daily basis that they were able to lose weight with relative ease – I watched as the crisis turned into an epidemic. The numbers continued to rise with dizzying speed: 27 million French citizens were overweight. The phenomenon seemed universal, borderless. As I watched the developments closely, I was struck by a number of points that I observed but couldn't yet understand.

The first point – the starting point for my reflection and my work – centred on the average birth weight of infants in the West. In the space of thirty years, from 1970 to 2000, this average underwent a startling increase.

In 1970, the average birth weight was 6.6 pounds; by 2000, the number had risen to 7.7 pounds. This neared the limit for what was considered overweight. Today, however, 7.7 pounds is the norm, and only an infant of 8.8 pounds or more is considered a big baby.

What explains this recent and significant increase in birth weight? We know that the foetus lives a completely passive life, depending solely on food from the mother. Scientifically and logically, then, the only possible explanation is a significant and global change in maternal nutrition. Pregnant women are actually eating less than they did in the past, but they are eating differently. Along with the rest of the population, their diet has been overtaken by an entirely new category of foods. This category consists of foods that have been industrially transformed, processed, concentrated and refined, becoming what we will call invasive carbohydrates. The term is meant to emphasise the lightning speed with which these carbohydrates are digested and assimilated.

The second point that caught my attention was the incomprehensible speed and amplitude of the explosion in overweight.

After starting slowly in the 1950s, the problem accelerated drastically in the 1970s, extending to affect **one quarter of the world's population in just forty years.** To my mind, there's no way such a progression can be explained by overeating and sedentary lifestyles, excessive calorie intake and under-exertion.

The third point is the appearance of type 2 diabetes in children and adolescents, a condition that previously affected only adults.

This aberrant phenomenon is strongest in developing countries, where food cultures have changed radically. Diabetes rates for children in China are reportedly four times higher than rates for children in the US (as per IASO)[2]. These rates mirror a sharp rise in obesity, which is affecting children at a younger and younger age. Who do we blame for the fact that one child in six is obese, or above all for the fact that the signs of this obesity can already be detected at the age of two or three? Accusing children at that age of overconsumption or inactivity would be nonsensical.

The fourth point is the increased prevalence of gestational diabetes.

---

[2] *Obesity Reviews,* 2016 from the International Association for the Study of Obesity (IASO)

Gestational diabetes is diabetes that first appears during a pregnancy, typically during the last trimester. We know that hormones secreted naturally by the placenta make insulin less effective – this is known as insulin resistance. This forces the pancreas to secrete more insulin for protection. The exertion can exhaust the pancreas and induce temporary diabetes.

In evolutionary terms, this phenomenon, related to fat storage, probably represented an advantage, offering protection for pregnancy during times of scarcity. But the flood of invasive and highly processed sugars in the modern diet (and therefore in the diet of pregnant women) exceeds the abilities of the pancreas to control blood sugar levels.

This is evidenced by the fact that the number of women affected by gestational diabetes varies according to country and culture. For instance, the prevalence of the condition in France today ranges from 6 to 10 per cent; in the US, however, where we know that the proportion of sugars consumed is higher, it can be as high as 18 per cent. The many consequences of gestational diabetes include the risk of the child's being born larger than is optimal, being more likely to become obese at the start of adulthood and more easily developing glucose intolerance, which can develop into diabetes.

Another point is the concept of 'diabesity' – a combination of diabetes and obesity – that emerged several years ago.

These two conditions were long considered distinct, until a common cause was finally discovered: extra insulin was produced by the pancreas to deal with the onslaught of invasive sugars.

These five points were perplexing. They seemed to be linked; but the relation between them was a mystery. This mystery troubled me for a long time. I needed to find the connection between them.

The chance to solve the mystery came when my patients' files were transferred to a digital format. The change made it possible to compare their data more extensively and in much greater detail.

Exploring the new database brought to light a link between my patients' dietary choices during pregnancy and the birth weight of their children. For patients whom I had monitored for long enough, there was also information on the evolution of the weight of their children through to adolescence. My findings contained nothing absolute, no clear conclusions, but they were enough to focus my attention on pregnancy.

Driven by curiosity, by the need to understand, I started researching epigenetics, a body of scientific knowledge that has been revolutionising the foundation of genetics. The explanatory power of epigenetics shattered the mystery and brought the shadowy problems I was grappling with into the stark light of day.

The epigenetics revolution

The genetic code is fundamentally unchangeable. Contrary to what has long been thought, however, it can be modified in its expression when it encounters new pressures from the environment in which it is deployed. This modification can involve facilitation or impedance, activation or deactivation, addition or subtraction.

The genetic code for our species has produced 8,000 successive generations of humans without interruption – as with all mammals, each new individual being carried in a mother's womb.

For the first 7,998 generations, born up until the years 1965 to 1970, maternal nourishment differed according to place and time. But at *no* point did it contain what we today call highly processed carbohydrates or refined sugars. US production and consumption of these foods began to soar in the 1950s; they have increased each year since, without exception.

Relying on epigenetic discoveries and advances, my hypothesis is based on the fact that this new type of food, which emerged in the 1970s, is not provided for in the genetic code of our species. It upsets the system. This disruption affects the target organ, the pancreas, and one of its endocrine secretions, insulin. When a pregnant woman relies on this kind of food in her diet, in the short or long term, it marks a major event in the fifty-six divisions of the genetic programme that guides the transformation of an egg into a newborn over the course of nine months.

When you take a genetic score that has no 'knowledge' of sugars and introduce a massive sugar intake, the resulting collision has an impact on the foetal pancreas, and can impair its development.

This is where epigenetics comes in, playing a role that has been ignored until just twenty years ago. Epigenetics modifies the genetic score of the pancreas to accelerate cellular proliferation, increasing its number of cells. This results in the pancreas secreting more insulin. The extra insulin transforms more glucose into fat, which increases the size of the foetus, so that it is larger than normal at birth. Not only will the infant be born bigger, they will also have a weakened pancreas, one that will remain vulnerable.

The role of the pancreas is to monitor and regulate blood glucose levels generated by foods containing carbohydrates. When this rate exceeds 1.4 grams per litre, there are risks for the eyes, heart, kidneys, brain and arteries of the lower limbs. To prevent these problems, the pancreas reacts by secreting insulin, which lowers the glucose level to around 1 gram, where it is perfectly tolerated. The pancreas and its insulin arsenal play this role throughout a person's life.

Up until the 1960s, processed foods containing carbohydrates were rarely encountered under normal living conditions. Pregnant women consumed very little of them; human infants were born weighing about 6.6 pounds and had a normal pancreas.

When a pregnant woman today eats modern foods (as the rest of us do), the pancreas of the foetus she carries will have to deal with the excess glucose in their shared blood *much too early*. This results in a vulnerability, manifested by a number of signs:

- The first is a higher than normal birth weight.
- The second is a persisting tendency to have excess weight during a lifetime: it may start right away, in childhood or adolescence, or later.
- The third is the early appearance of a progressive loss of insulin sensitivity, known as insulin resistance.

From there, obesity, metabolic syndrome and diabetes may develop.

It is to counter this threat that I created the plan presented in this book – to help you avoid this result, which is as dangerous as it is *avoidable*.

You'll be surprised at how easy the measures are that form the basis of this plan, and how little frustration and privation is involved. Better still, your maternal instincts will bloom as you take the opportunity to give your child the best possible gift: a future.

BUT FOR THIS TO HAPPEN, YOU NEED TO BE CONVINCED.

I have written this book to share my firm beliefs on this subject. Each chapter is like a step on a ladder, and together they form a complete plan.

It's important to note that this plan has its roots firmly embedded in an immense body of collective scientific work. Hundreds of thousands of scientific studies, surveys, research projects and observations from every continent were directly or indirectly taken into account to ensure that this plan is sound.

Chapters 2, 3 and 4 focus on the enemy: excess weight, obesity and diabetes, and the unnecessary sugars we eat. It is essential to recognise the seriousness of the problem. These chapters set the stage for the rest of the book, which will give you the means to avoid these risks for your unborn child over the course of your pregnancy.

All too often we talk about the fact of weight problems without discussing the reasons for them. Thus, these chapters focus on the deep and hidden causes of this condition: its physical, mental and social components.

'I eat because I feel bad – the worse I feel, the more sugar I eat.'

'I feel bad because my life seems out of control. There's so much going on in the world, so much to take in, but I feel trapped, and the reward centres in my brain aren't satisfied by the stimulation I'm getting.'

Chapter 5 is devoted to the central actor in the plan: the pancreas – your own adult pancreas, but even more importantly, the pancreas of the unborn child you are carrying, which is developing with each passing day.

I have already said that the explosion of this crisis cannot be explained solely by overeating and a sedentary lifestyle. These two causes alone could never lead to an epidemic of this proportion. In my view, the scope of the crisis is related to the arrival of a generation of newborns whose pancreas has been left *vulnerable*, which leads to an exponential increase in the number of individuals affected.

To understand my plan and to be able to follow it, you

will need to understand how this unique organ functions and develops.

Chapter 6 focuses on our species and the genetic code that expresses it. Every known species has a genetic code containing alimentary inclinations and instructions that affect nutrition, physiology and behaviour. What foods are universal to humans? Which foods have always been a part of our lives, and which ones are rarer? And most important, which foods were never a part of our lives and might pose a risk of disrupting our biological makeup?

Chapters 7 and 8 focus on the centrepiece of my demonstration, *the science of epigenetics.* With its boldness and amazing explanatory power, epigenetics has captivated the international scientific community, myself included. I will attempt to share it with you in all its simplicity. Your best allies will be your maternal instinct and common sense; they're enough to make you a receptive audience. Understanding and accepting the simple and coherent message in this chapter will lead directly to benefits: for the child you're carrying and, in the long term, for you.

My aim is to take advantage of the intellectual openness and clear-sightedness you possess as a pregnant woman to pass on one main lesson.

This lesson rests entirely on a single fact: that invasive processed sugars are not naturally human foods, and that there is a sugar even worse than white sugar, one that is more invasive, quicker to pass through the digestive system, requiring more insulin: processed white flour.

There is a world of difference between modern-day white flour and the flour that was used fifty years ago – between white flour and whole flour. It's important to realise that whole-wheat flour is *supplemented*: it is basically white flour to which wheat bran has been added. As soon as it reaches the stomach, the mixture comes apart. The white flour is processed much more quickly than the wheat, reaching the blood much faster and in larger doses. In other words, whole-wheat bread ultimately behaves similarly to white bread. It's akin to the world of difference between fruit juice and whole fruits.

In the final chapter, I offer guidance on how to practise the plan. You'll be surprised how simple the measures are. In no time at all, you'll be speeding towards victory.

To conclude my introduction to this book, I would like to offer a promise and an absolute commitment. Not a single one of the dietary measures in this plan will disadvantage you or cause any risk – for you and much less for your unborn child. Each step will be nothing but beneficial to the health of you both.

CHAPTER 2

The Enemy: Excess Weight, Obesity and Diabetes

The risks, dangers and menaces

What you should know to protect the child you're bringing into the world

The weight crisis has progressed with incredible speed and generated untold harm. We can't go on excusing it as just a symptom of women's *joie de vivre*, the result of a happy and carefree lifestyle. Excess weight has become a terribly efficient killer – indeed, it's the leading health risk threatening us today.

Obesity is a recent condition

Excess weight problems existed before 1944, but only a small portion of the population was affected. Being heavy or even obese was seen as a visible sign of wealth and power. It meant prominence, in the most literal sense of the word.

In pre-war France, it was estimated that 100,000 people were overweight or obese. By 1960, there were over a million.

In 2009, 27 million people were overweight; 7 million of these were obese. The lifespan of the obese was *nine years* shorter. And in fact, France was more successful than most countries at resisting the epidemic. If France had the same proportion of overweight people as the US has, obesity numbers would be twice what they are now.

What explains this phenomenon? How is it related to our historical moment, and how has it progressed?

The usual explanation for the weight crisis is simple: it is caused by caloric intake exceeding energy expenditure. Unfortunately, the answer adds nothing to our understanding. It offers us the *how* of the weight crisis, but not the *why*.

So now let's ask why.

The goal of this book is to show – in a demonstrable, scientific way – that if you are nurturing an unborn child in your womb, *you have the power to take decisive action for your child's future weight*. And if all the mothers in the world shared that understanding and were aware of the simple measures that followed from it, it would be possible to stop the progression of the weight crisis – even to reverse it.

That claim might seem bold – even utopic. How could

we even conceive of stopping the scourge so easily, one that has already caused *tens of millions of deaths around the world*? No country on Earth has been able to do so.

The objections are understandable. I've spent three full years working on this project, and I haven't worked alone. I've spoken with dozens of committed scientists who specialise in this area, and analysed thousands of studies on the subject.

There's no disputing the fact that, ever since our species came into being some 200,000 years ago, the transmission of life from a mother-to-be to her unborn child has mainly taken place in a *stable dietary context*, despite cultural and geographic variations. This context has respected the nutrition needs specific to humans.

Yet, since the middle of the last century, this diet has collapsed. That collapse has been simultaneous with the weight crisis. The imbalance that now exists is due to the industrialisation of human food production. Food has become merchandise. As such, it is subject to the usual demands of cost reduction and productivity. The priority is profit, with no regard for the nutritional consequences.

The industries based on the intensive production of sugar, flour and their derivatives are making their fortunes by making us fat, from when we are born until our middle age.

Then, in our golden years, the pharmaceutical industry profits by selling us treatments for the health problems caused by excess weight.

Our societies are governed by economics. Thus, the lobbies for these industries have created a defensive shell of disinformation to protect their interests. Governments and public health bodies may not even really want to win the war against excess weight; there are too many private and public interests at stake. That's why we hear double talk from decision-makers who condemn the epidemic but offer no solutions – or, worse, who propose poor solutions that are doomed to fail.

Do we have to throw up our hands in defeat? No. I developed the plan contained in this book to address these enormous obstacles. I want to offer a new path. Consumer culture, the cause of weight problems, undermines all of our attempts to remedy them, no matter how much suffering they cause. That means the problem must be approached differently: it must be tackled at the root. We must prevent excess weight from developing in the first place.

The reason I'm addressing you through this book is that the power to stop the deadly epidemic is in your hands. You are preparing to create new life. During part of your pregnancy, your life will be affected by maternal hormones. These are the same hormones that, for time immemorial, have radically transformed women, for a certain number of months, into a new being: a potential mother – and importantly, in today's context, a mother rather than a consumer.

I'm addressing you directly because I believe that, during this period of grace, the siren call of consumption will be drowned out by the instinct to care for the child in your womb. By the end of the book, my argument will be complete and clear. You'll be fully convinced, I believe, that my project is concrete and that my reasoning is sound. I'll show you how you can actively protect your unborn child during their primary development, and prevent them from forming a vulnerability that will accompany them for the rest of their life.

If you're pregnant, you probably already know that adult nutrition differs from child nutrition, and even more so from that of a newborn. But the difference is greater still when it comes to a foetus undergoing intensive development.

During the months of your pregnancy, you have to pay close attention to the information you take in, particularly when it comes to advertising messages. **The gatekeepers for advertising rate the truth and risks of messages about food products according to their consumption by *adults*, and do not consider their *effect on an unborn child* carried by an adult woman.**

One of the main objectives of this book is to show you that the primary cause of obesity and diabetes in adults – which in turn are the leading causes of mortality today – is sugars, and the insulin that controls blood sugar levels.

While it takes decades for sugars to profoundly affect an adult's health, this is not the case for a growing foetus. As the foetus incorporates the diet of the woman who carries it, its developing pancreas is at risk of being disrupted at a crucial moment. This will cause a *vulnerability* that will make the risks from sugars greater and potentially more harmful.

I created this plan because I am convinced that the unbelievable explosion in excess weight around the world is in large part due to the rise in the number of children who are affected by a vulnerability to weight problems and diabetes that they acquired in their mother's womb. This vulnerability remains when these children grow up and become adults. A diet too high in refined sugars has generated a new model of human being: one that is infinitely more prone to gaining weight and becoming diabetic. It's this process that helps explain how the population of overweight people has risen from several hundred million to over 2 billion.

In 1980, there were 100 million diabetics in the world; in under two generations, the number has soared to more than 400 million.

If you are pregnant, you are the sole link between what you put in your mouth and the glucose that ends up in the blood and pancreas of your child. Therefore, you are naturally the only person who can ensure your child's dietary protection. And you can ensure this protection only if you understand the necessity of avoiding glucose-related problems and know how to avoid them. My mission is to help you become aware of that necessity and give you the right tools to succeed.

The food production industry and its powerful army

of advertisers don't set out to wilfully harm anyone. But they are driven by a single objective: to produce profit as efficiently as possible. That's why it's crucial that during the space of several months, when our species gives you the singular mission of bearing and bringing forth life, you must learn to distinguish foods that are tolerable for you but not for your child. It isn't easy to maintain a critical stance while watching highly seductive television commercials. You need to stay on guard during the months of pregnancy.

It's common for a commercial to convince you that you really want a biscuit – not just a sugary biscuit, but one that's also loaded with flour. Somewhere inside you, you think you need that snack to stay alert and compensate for the energy you've lost over the morning. But your maternal instinct will probably alert you correctly: it's a trap. That same instinct will keep you from falling into that trap. To take just one example, one of the best-selling biscuits in France is 62 per cent carbohydrates, and almost 20 per cent white sugar. And yet, incredibly, this biscuit is presented as weight-loss friendly.

Before writing this book, I spent a lot of time reflecting. I was reluctant to join in this struggle; I've had sufficient experience with lobbies to know how powerful they are, and to know that this project will be much more a target for attack than my diet was. That's because this project tackles the problem at the roots. It therefore poses a serious threat to the activities and the profits of a very powerful industry.

My hope is that the more the epidemic spreads, the more

costly and alienating it becomes, the more consumers will rise up to form a resistance against the suffering it causes. The day will come when the producers learn that their economic model has sprung a leak, and that their own survival depends on shifting the paradigm. The process is already under way. In 2014, annual sales for The Coca-Cola Company and McDonald's actually declined. (Coca-Cola dropped 1.37 per cent to reach $12.57 billion: a far cry from the $12.87 billion expected. McDonald's had a similar result, with sales of $7.18 billion, lower than the $7.29 billion anticipated.)

But this evolution may take time. We should take any strategy available to us that can speed up the process, one that I believe is inevitable – especially in light of the fact that, somewhere in the world, one overweight, obese or diabetic person dies *each second.*

In the attack I will mount in this book, I have an ally – a very powerful ally. This ally is implanted in the heart of every human – indeed, every mammal. It's the maternal instinct. I've witnessed enough women quit smoking, drinking or smoking marijuana without hesitation upon learning that they are pregnant. I'm convinced that, if I can pass on my beliefs and the results of my research, all the lobbies combined couldn't hide the truth – period.

But now let's return to the dangers of being overweight, its consequences and complications. The aim is not to scare you, but simply to describe the enemy from every angle. And it's important to remember one thing: weight problems are *as dangerous as they are avoidable*.

Complications resulting from excess weight and obesity

The consequences are many: they are linked with a vast range of pathologies. Quite simply, an obese person is ten times more at risk of having a weight-related disease than a non-obese person.

Type 2 diabetes

This section will be of particular interest to you if there are diabetics in your family, you're seriously overweight, you have previously suffered from gestational diabetes, or you eat a lot of sugary foods or very fast carbohydrates such as white bread, white rice, white pasta or potatoes.

Diabetes is by far the most direct complication from being overweight. This has led to its being grouped under a broad new category: diabesity. The concept was created because obesity and diabetes have the same origin: both are caused by insulin and the pancreas that secretes it. The vast majority of type 2 diabetics are overweight or obese.

The danger of diabetes lies in the fact that it's a silent condition that emerges once the damage – which often comes in multiple forms – already poses a serious threat.

Diabetes emerges when the pancreas loses control of glucose concentration in the blood. At around 100 mg/dl, glucose is necessary – indispensable, in fact. But beyond

115 mg/dl, it becomes increasingly corrosive for many organs. At a fasting glucose of 126 mg/dl, diabetes is already present.

If it weren't for the pancreas, however – if we didn't have insulin – glucose would be deadly from about 700 to 1,000 mg/dl. A diabetic whose pancreas has shut down and who is taking insulin and forgets to take their treatment would go into a diabetic coma and die in less than an hour just from consuming half a French bread and a fizzy drink.

What are the complications of diabetes?

Heart attack

Heart attacks strike diabetics three to four times more often than non-diabetics. Diabetic heart attack is often silent, since nerve damage reduces the sensation of pain, which means that diagnosis and treatment tend to be delayed. In the acute phase of a heart attack, insulin is injected to lower the amount of blood sugar attacking the heart; the gravity of having too much glucose is all too clear.

Blindness

Diabetes is the leading cause of acquired blindness. A prolonged excess of glucose in the blood CARAMELISES the small capillaries and arterioles that deliver nutrients to the retina. This causes oedema, dilation and bleeding, which eventually lead to blindness.

Once again, glucose is the culprit. And, as always, high

glucose levels are caused by failure of the pancreas and its resulting inability to secrete insulin.

Arterial hypertension

This condition is so commonly associated with diabetes that it's almost considered an inherent symptom. Arterial hypertension affects one out of two diabetics. This condition, in combination with excess weight localised on the paunch and diabetes, sets the stage for metabolic syndrome.

Hypertension worsens the prognosis of diabetes by accelerating the onset of heart attack and especially stroke.

Kidney damage

Sugar is the most common and most damaging toxin for the kidneys; and diabetes is the number-one cause of kidney failure, which requires sufferers to use a dialysis machine to rid the body of its waste.

We often hear that proteins damage the kidneys. This unfounded rumour is just a diversion used by the sugar industry. It's meant to distract us from the fact that the only nutrient that alters the kidneys is sugar, when blood glucose levels exceed 140 mg/dl.

Naturopathy

Nerve damage from sugar is one of the most common complications from diabetes. It occurs when prolonged excess of glucose attacks the nerves and profoundly impairs their functioning. One of the worst and most common problems is its effect on sensitivity to pain. Intense pain can be caused merely by contact between a piece of cloth and the foot; or numbness can result that makes sufferers unaware that they're being burned or injured. This explains why many infected wounds suffered by diabetics end up requiring amputation. Reduced sugar consumption and glycaemic control (control of blood sugar) can diminish this complication if the onset is recent. If it's not, controlling sugar can only stabilise the condition.

Diabetes and amputation

When diabetes is managed poorly over a long period of time, atherosclerosis may occur. The condition results in less oxygen-rich arterial blood reaching the extremities. Just a tiny wound, recognised too late due to a loss of sensitivity, can lead to infections that don't heal. Atherosclerosis is a breeding ground for small gangrenes of the big toe, the foot and to some extent the leg. **Seventy per cent of non-accidental amputations are caused by diabetes.**

Diabetes and male erection

Diabetes is the leading organic cause of erectile dysfunction. Between 50 and 75 per cent of diabetic men lose their ability to maintain erection and suffer from sexual problems.

A normal erection is caused by blood being trapped in the cavernous tissue of the penis. For a sufficient and sustainable erection, it is essential that the arteries, veins, nerves and male hormones play their role perfectly.

With diabetics, however, high glucose levels damage the arterial, venous and nervous systems. Furthermore, being overweight encourages the conversion of male hormones – testosterone – into female hormones – oestrogen. When diabetes reaches the complications stage, it becomes a nightmarish condition: everything starts to break down simultaneously. The mounting problems often lead to a state of depression, which, combined with erectile dysfunction, can cause relationship problems for couples.

Sleep apnoea

Sleep apnoea is pauses in breathing that occur during deep sleep: breathing stops for more than ten seconds, more than five times an hour. These apnoeas have a profound effect on quality of life, causing debilitating fatigue, headaches and drowsiness in a waking state.

In obese patients, weight gain particularly affects the base of the tongue, which is very rich in adipose tissue. The increased weight of the tongue puts pressure on the larynx, reducing its diameter to the point of obstruction. Sleep apnoea sufferers often experience slackening and loss of muscle tone in the throat and larynx, which aggravates the obstruction.

Joint pain

Excess weight puts mechanical stress on cartilage, wearing

it out faster. The most sensitive joints and those most often affected are the knees, as well as the lumbar vertebrae, and, for those who are predisposed, the hips. Before resorting to drug therapy or surgery, rheumatologists and orthopaedic surgeons ask their patients to lose weight. Patients tend to comply, since losing weight quickly improves symptoms.

When diabetes is a factor, other symptoms appear that tend to be misdiagnosed. The increase in glucose damages and weakens the tendons. In combination with their excess weight, diabetics suffer from multiple tendonitis problems that disrupt their motor skills and cause night pain that affects quality of sleep.

Alzheimer's or type 3 diabetes

Diabetes increases the risk of developing Alzheimer's greatly – by 1.5 to 2 times. Toxicity from excess sugar in the blood also affects the brain. The extra glucose attacks microcirculation and alters the neurons. Furthermore, resistance to insulin leads to inflammatory stress, which adds to the effects on nerve cells. Finally, the body neutralises the excess glucose by transforming it into triglycerides, which contribute to neurons being damaged by amyloid plaques.

All Alzheimer's specialists today believe that a diet low in sugar, along with physical activity that consumes glucose, delays the onset of the disease.

You're probably beginning to see that, as we explore the different complications caused by excess weight, the same culprits keep popping up: excess sugar, and our body's attempts to fend off its toxicity with insulin and the pancreas that secretes it.

At some point, we are forced to confront a number of questions.

- Why, in a growing number of humans over the span of two generations, is the pancreas unable to perform its functions?
- Why are more and more babies born bigger than in the past, again over the span of two generations?
- Why are diabetes rates going up among obese people?
- Why are more women today affected by gestational diabetes than in their grandmothers' time?
- Why are children and adolescents today becoming diabetic, when two generations ago diabetes affected only middle-aged adults?

All these questions point to a category of foods that appeared quite recently: foods that exceed the physiological abilities of our pancreas. We don't need to look far. Foods rich in proteins (meats, fish, etc.) and foods rich in fats (oils and butter) haven't changed much. Carbohydrates, however, have become ubiquitous.

And, in particular, carbohydrates that have been modified and processed by the food industry are to blame. Each 'step forward' in industrial processing makes them more penetrating, invasive and immediate. When they flood the bloodstream, they abruptly raise blood glucose levels, requiring the pancreas to secrete ever more insulin. Insulin in turn 'makes you fat' by transforming glucose into fat. The pancreas, being overworked, can eventually become exhausted, which opens the door to diabetes.

Only a very strong pancreas can deal with such aggressive and artificial foods. This strength is developed during the last six months over pregnancy. To achieve it, it is essential that the foetus's tiny pancreas, which develops so rapidly, be given the chance to grow without being bombarded by an excessive amount of these foods.

My goal can be boiled down to this: I want to convince you to eat the way people ate only two generations ago. And I particularly want you to do so during the fourth and fifth months of your pregnancy – the most decisive months for the development of the pancreas of the child you're carrying.

The heart

The heart is one of the target organs for excess weight.

First, in people suffering from obesity, the exertion required for the heart to pump is directly correlated to the amount of excess weight a person has. Carrying just a 20 lb backpack can raise the rate and increase the strength of cardiac contraction in an individual who is unfit.

Second, excess fat creates a resistance to blood flow. More fat means the heart muscle has to pump harder to get through areas where fat is concentrated. This creates an increase in blood pressure.

In the arteries, obesity and diabetes are very often related to high triglycerides and 'bad' blood cholesterol, as well as lower 'good cholesterol'. The combined effect of the problems is clogging of the arteries and weakening of their walls.

The combination of narrowed arteries weakened by atherosclerotic plaques and blood circulating under high pressure creates the conditions for dangerous circulatory events in areas where vascularisation is essential. One example would be the coronary arteries, which deliver nutrients to the heart; the closing of these arteries causes angina and heart attack.

Stroke

Once again, the same causes are at play, but in this case, high blood pressure plays a leading role. In obese individuals and diabetics, the large carotid arteries that reach up the neck to carry blood to the brain often become partially obstructed. The same goes for the entire cerebral arterial system. Under these strenuous conditions, all it takes is poorly managed or ignored hypertension (high blood pressure) for an artery to become blocked, or, worse, ruptured, to cause bleeding and compression of the brain.

Cancer

Today we have total scientific consensus on the direct links between cancer and diet. According to a European anti-cancer organisation, almost half a million new cases of cancer among adults worldwide can be attributed to excess weight and obesity. Among the known factors, one of the most common is excess weight and diabetes.[3]

We know that sugar and invasive carbohydrates end up in the blood in the form of glucose; and we know that glucose plays a key role in the development and propagation of cancer. But how does this occur?

Let's compare a normal cell and a cancerous cell. A normal cell functions in a hybrid mode: its nutrients are glucose and fatty acids (from sugar or fat). A cancerous cell, however, doesn't use fat. **Its sole nutrient is glucose, which it needs to survive.**

However, glucose does more than just fuel the multiplication and dissemination of cancerous cells. It also causes the reflexive production of insulin, which indirectly triggers the production of insulin-like growth factor (IGF) – a powerful protein that stimulates the growth of cancerous cells. Finally (as if all that wasn't enough), we know that hypertrophic fat cells in overweight or obese people experience stress and produce cytokines, which create inflammation.

For all these reasons, most oncologists today recommend to their patients a diet **low in invasive sugars**, which slows down tumour development and especially metastasis, the spread of cancer.

---

[3] 'The key statistics of cancers', www.ligue-cancer.net/article/6397_les-chiffres-cles-des-cancers

Depression

Obesity and diabetes are now recognised as twin conditions; they fall under the new concept of diabesity. Combined, the two conditions commonly lead to dissatisfaction, suffering and anxiety. These in turn are statistically closely linked with a third condition, one that is also spreading rapidly: depression.

A very large study showed that diabetics are twice as likely to suffer from depression as non-diabetics.[4] The association has more to do with the psychological impact of the disease than with its metabolic factors. The proof: **undiagnosed diabetics or those unaware of their condition are less likely to be depressed than those who are aware.**

As for excess weight, a large study by a Netherlands university found that obesity promotes depression, and depression in turn leads to weight gain.[5] Specifically, obese individuals have an almost 55 per cent risk of developing depression, and people suffering from depression have a 58 per cent risk of becoming obese.

The accumulation of excess weight, especially when it reaches the obesity stage, can create a feeling of exclusion and lack of self-worth. The sense of rejecting one's body and self-image, and the feeling (real or imagined) of being

---

[4] Anderson, R.J., Freedland, K.E., Clouse R.E. and Lustman, P.J., *The Prevalence of Comorbid Depression in Adults with Diabetes, Diabet. Med.*, Nov. 23 2006, 23 (11): 1165-73

[5] Luppino, F.S., det Wit, L.M., et al, 'Overweight, obesity and depression: a systematic review and meta-analysis of longitudinal studies', *Arch. Gen. Psychiatry*, March 2010, 67 (3), p 220-9

discriminated against, can lead to complexes, inhibition and loss of self-esteem.

Then there's the flip side of the coin. People with depression tend to feel a desperate need for satisfaction. They tend to find this satisfaction in sugary and fatty foods, which cause weight gain.

Depression also diminishes a person's motivation to stick to a diet programme or diabetes management regime, just as it impairs compliance with medication and especially physical activity.

Finally, to make matters worse, most antidepressants cause weight gain.

The butterfly effect

In this chapter, I have tried to present the enemy in its true form. The enemy has a special power: those who suffer from it or are threatened believe – with good reason – that they can evade the threat at any moment. They can therefore wait till another day to make a change. But delaying can lead to dire results. The same goes for tobacco.

But there's reason for optimism. Most smokers quit when they learn they're pregnant. And the plan I'm proposing here is infinitely simpler than giving up tobacco.

The enemy – excess weight, obesity and diabetes – has already attacked more than 2 million humans. And the monumental amount of suffering and hardship it has caused is a recent phenomenon. For reasons I will explain in the next chapter, we know exactly when the crisis was born: 1944.

Determining a birth date for the worldwide phenomenon means finding an explanation, even making a diagnosis. In 1944, something new appeared, so significant that it would deeply change humanity's lifestyle – and thus its physical and mental health. The event marked the shift to a new model of civilisation: humanity moved to a system governed by economics. This system carried an obligation for its members to consume more and more each year.

All attempts to fight excess weight since then have failed. Rational and effective strategies are rightly perceived by food producers as a threat to their interests. Understandably, therefore, these producers fight them with every means at their disposal.

The struggle before us means resisting the hurricane of packaging that has swept up our civilisation. But every hurricane starts as a gentle breeze. It brings to mind the well-known question:

Does the flap of a butterfly's wings in Brazil set off a tornado in Texas?

In other words, where does the problem start? My belief, and the basis for the project undertaken in this book, is that this question offers us a real solution. If it's true that the flap of a butterfly's wings can stir up a hurricane, then we also have a way to prevent the storm: we start at that original movement.

For readers who are at the start of a pregnancy, it is time for you to change the weather. That's what it will take to prevent your child from being born in a hurricane that leaves weight problems and diabetes in its wake.

CHAPTER 3

Excess Weight, Obesity and Diabetes: How and Why

What every mother-to-be should know about the reasons for excess weight, to protect her child

Five little-known reasons for the crisis in excess weight, obesity and diabetes

1) Excess weight and obesity aren't a focus in the medical field; they are not confronted and taken seriously by physicians until they reach the complications stage. So long as excess weight does not threaten life or health, it is seen as a trivial matter, a subject for magazines and fitness gurus. Unfortunately, however, when the complications arise, they are serious and difficult to reverse.

2) Excess weight is a result of the intersection of supply and demand.

On one side is the compulsive craving for foods that provide quick gratification. This craving arises because we want to make up for deficiencies and frustrations in other areas of our life.

On the other side is an overabundant supply of food – an ever-expanding selection of appealing and seductive products. People who become overweight suffer as their bodies change; but the suffering seems minor compared with the suffering they would experience if they deprived themselves of the weight-causing products.

3) The invasion of industrially produced, highly processed carbohydrates. These modern foods are encountered by a pancreas that came into being in a time before it could be designed or programmed to deal with them.

When the glucose in your blood rises from 100 mg/dl to just 200 mg/dl, the blood becomes seriously toxic to all the organs it irrigates. As a response, this blood sugar is transformed into fat, which leads to excess weight and eventually diabetes.

4) The fourth explanation for the crisis is the logic of the market.

Producers that control food supplies have only one objective: to convince consumers to buy their products. They have two ways of achieving this. The first employs the classic logic of seduction and competition through marketing, packaging and advertising. The second is infinitely more insidious. It focuses on undermining the natural foundations for human happiness: family fulfilment, love and sexuality, the use of the body, spending time in nature, spirituality: all simple pleasures that don't cost a thing. When it comes to choosing between happiness and the need to have consumers buying a product, the result is inevitable. A well-established sociological law, widely put into practice in our age, tells us that *unhappy consumers consume more than happy consumers.*

But this same market logic also offers hope. Industry profits depend on our playing our role as consumers. If we vote with our wallets and insist that we want and need healthful food products, the industry will respond. It will design, develop and promote the products we want.

But, for that to happen, it's crucial that opinion leaders, health authorities, media and politicians believe in this cause, and declare their support. Producers are savvy: they know that products with good nutritional content will eventually become their El Dorado. They're just waiting for a clear signal that it's time to jump into the ring. They've already demonstrated this willingness by offering diet drinks, sugar-free chewing gum and, more recently, gluten-free products.

5) The fifth reason is crucial, since it's at the origin of the crisis. It's the first beating of the butterfly's wings, so to

speak. And it is the target of this book: the determining role of maternal nutrition on the pancreas of an unborn child.

The weight crisis: a recent struggle between the individual and society

We are about to enter a subject area that should be of interest to everyone – but especially to mothers-to-be, who are in the process of learning how to give life to a new generation. Strap on your seat belt.

Let's begin with a metaphor: the bee and the hive.

Imagine a bee that gathers nectar, letting its path be guided by the scents and colours of various flowers. The bee leaves its home, the hive, to forage, burrowing into the corollas of flowers so it can find the pollen and nectar they conceal. Eventually, guided by the sun, it returns to the hive. There it deposits what will later become honey and wax.

But if the hive belongs to a human – specifically a honey producer – the honey and wax end up being diverted from their primary function. And if the bees live near a refinery that treats cane sugar, they cannot visit flowers or collect their pollen.

Now let's consider the human hive. It's worth your time: by the end of this chapter, you will look at life differently. When you encounter an idea that changes your view fundamentally, there's no turning back.

We will look at two inseparable and complementary sides of our human world: the individual (namely, you) and society (the one in which you live). Each has its own programme to follow. But it is the recent opposition between the two – between the individual and society – that is at the origin of weight problems and decreased happiness.

The primary role of the individual

Consider any human – yourself, for instance. At a very early stage of your life, during the first months *in utero*, an initial command is issued within the hypothalamus – one of the deepest and most archaic parts of the brain, a part we share with reptiles. If life were compared to an ultra-sophisticated computer program, this command would be the first and fundamental rule of the program.

That command is: 'Live'.

Let's give that transmitter another name: the Life Pulsar. The Life Pulsar could be compared to an embryo's heart, which starts to beat at around the same period. The Pulsar transmits the simple need or appetite for life. It's what makes you get up every morning, without questioning the instinct, to enjoy the world and build a life for yourself. Like hunger or thirst or sexual desire, the will to live is driven by energy, desire, motivation – and it moves you more powerfully when you're preparing to bring new life into the world.

This motivating energy naturally flows into different channels, resulting in a number of behaviours being expressed. These behaviours are very familiar to each of us: their job is to keep us alive. Neurologists call them reward-seeking behaviours.

I believe that this reward system is probably one of the keys to the evolution of life; and the system probably became part of the evolution of our species at its very origins. Incredibly simple and amazingly effective, it has persisted over countless generations and is still very present today. **The more useful a behaviour is for the protection and perpetuation of life, the more reward it earns; the more reward it earns, the more the behaviour is desirable and practiced.**

But it goes even further. Behaviours that are favourable to a given species are selected and integrated into its very DNA. The first of these behaviours is centred on the need to feed oneself. This need is a condition for existence – without it, everything quickly grinds to a halt. The benefit is big, and hence the reward is, too.

But the intensity of this need varies from person to person. On rare occasions, I've encountered patients who, while not anorexic, don't experience the drive to eat. These individuals take in nourishment only in order to survive.

The same thing happens with sexual desire – a need associated with love, the pleasure of giving life and protecting it, and which provides a major reward. A widespread repulsion towards sex would spell the end of our species.

And reward and the circuits through which it is provided are not limited to these two needs. During my professional life, I've met with patients who are unable to switch off their exacerbated need to eat; in monitoring these patients,

I discovered that they had difficulty satisfying other human needs, and that they compensated for their dissatisfaction by eating more food as a reward.

I followed this line of investigation further. My work was guided by considering the lives of early man and the last Neanderthals, and even the great apes. My goal was essentially to identify and understand our reasons for living.

In this way, I was gradually able to identify ten fundamental needs that are inscribed in the human genetic code – our DNA. These needs encapsulate the wisdom of our bodies and our behaviours that ensure life and survival. Satisfying these needs gives us rewards; it provides a beneficial and fulfilling experience. There are exactly ten of these needs – not one more, despite all the research I have done, which continues to this day. These are the basis for my theory of the *ten pillars of happiness*, which you'll find on **pages 56–78**.

Let's return now to the question of the function of the individual, mentioned earlier. This function forms a loop: it starts with the Life Pulsar, and returns to it.

The Life Pulsar, as the name suggests, is a source of motivation, will, appetite and magnetism. Like a homing device, this pulse takes on the behaviour of the reward that best suits it.

Our genes, the start of our childhood, the culture that surrounds us, our place and our moment in history, encounters we have with others: all these result in some of our reward channels opening up, while others are narrowed or completely closed off. It is not necessary to use all our reward channels in order to live, to be a human who experiences biological rewards; we can function with just three or four.

When a reward-seeking behaviour is successful, the reward appears. This is manifested at two levels simultaneously.

The first is something we experience on a daily basis. It's the sense of enjoying life, of experiencing good feelings – from simple contentment to pleasure to euphoria or joy – and the unfurling of energy that results, the kind that makes you leap for joy and cry out with happiness.

The second is located at a deeper level; it is strictly biological, and functions unconsciously. The reward is expressed by an intracerebral secretion of two chemical mediators: dopamine and serotonin. The primary function of these two substances is to return to the Life Pulsar – to recharge it, so to speak.

The energy that was emitted thus ends up back at the beginning of the circuit. These two chemical mediators are commonly cited to explain dependence and addiction.

So, in summary: the Life Pulsar emits energy that activates the reward circuits. This releases dopamine and serotonin, which closes the circuit by making their return to the Pulsar for recharging.

It's this circuit that keeps human life going.

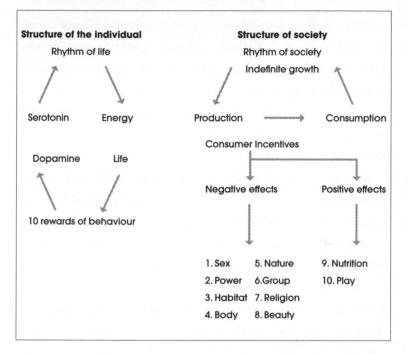

The primary role of society

Human society consists of a group of individuals living and working together. It could be compared to a human body: like cells, individuals cooperate to form the social body.

During the very long period when humankind lived as hunter-gatherers, human societies were made up of 50 to 200 people. With the emergence of civilisation, societies became progressively larger, eventually expanding to include millions of people.

A society obviously doesn't have the same physical embodiment as an individual, but it is governed by analogous rules.

Like the individual, society is driven by its own 'Pulsar'. In this respect, there's a difference between the social body and an individual's body: the Social Pulsar is not a fixed part of our genetic framework. It can be altered.

That's what happened in 1944, when a cultural revolution introduced a radically new pulsar. This change resulted in a new model of civilisation, one that deeply uprooted society and the lives and development of its members.

In that year, at the end of the war, the shaken allied countries gathered, at the invitation of the United States, in Bretton Woods, a small town in New Hampshire, to implement a new social model. The objective was to rebuild their economies.

It was in this context of rebuilding that the concept of indefinite growth was born. The trials of the war and feats of technology instilled a powerful hope for prosperity and happiness. The concept of permanent growth was born from this hope. This concept became the foundation of our societies – it was the social equivalent of the Life Pulsar for the individual.

The primary command of the Individual Pulsar is *live*; that of society is *grow indefinitely, and more each year.*

A growing society is one that creates more wealth, goods, objects and services than the previous year. But to produce more upstream, it is necessary that there are consumers downstream who will absorb the surplus produced.

It was a totally new model: one that became known as the consumer society.

So long as it was a matter of meeting basic human needs, the opportunity for this consumption was considered a blessing. Human society welcomed elevators, vehicles, new medications and means of communication; intense physical effort was gradually eradicated.

Once the more basic needs were covered, other comfort-providing products appeared – appliances, washing machines and dishwashers, and many more – all of which were equally welcomed.

Eventually, consumers started to feel that their needs were met. They were ready to take a relaxed breath from consuming. But this threatened to disrupt the system.

To maintain the rate of consumption – household demand, as it is famously known – society flew to the rescue of the great production machine. The solution was to develop two types of incentives that would push consumer temptation to new levels.

One, a positive incentive: the classical component of selling a product, based on cosmetic seduction. Marketing, packaging, advertising, 'As Seen on TV': all these come together and form a collective attack to promote impulse buys.

Two, a negative incentive: a deeply immoral one, which aims to do nothing less than distance individuals from the satisfaction of the **ten major needs**, those that are most natural and human, in order to push them towards consumption instead.

Why?

Of those ten natural needs, eight are free. Consider the powerful need covered by the term 'sexuality', most broadly speaking, which includes love and family. Loving one's wife, mother or children is basic, natural and powerful; and it does not involve consumption. The consumption industry aligns itself with anything that can break the hold of these fundamental needs.

Two of these ten needs are natural and can also be profitable: the need for food and the need for play.

Food products sell extremely well, since they provide a sensory experience and have been made addictive with the inclusion of processed ingredients.

Play and recreation is another deeply human need: the joy of having fun, laughing, dancing and singing with other humans. This need for play has been diverted from its primary function to become an object of consumption. Today it is solitary and passive, delivered by TV screens, electronic games and entertainment on demand. It sells extremely well.

For fifty years, the engagement between our hearts and the world around us has been quietly and progressively eroded. It took decades for us to forget the smell of trees, to eradicate physical effort, to relegate beauty to walled-in museums, to encase spirituality in steel and concrete, to restrict the pleasure of rewarding work to a lucky elite, to turn the intense need to belong to a group into consumer individualism, whose pleasures are wrapped in a plastic package.

It's worth asking who is behind this profound attack on humankind. Is there one man or some devious group somewhere out there that is responsible for such a policy?

The simple answer is no. The shift is a result of a structural change to our place in the world. With the vastness and complexity of an overpopulated planet in which life expectancy has doubled, a new society has emerged. This society has come to dominate the individual in order to achieve massification: maximum sales growth.

This new society depends on the economy and technology for its survival. As the great social machine turns, its fundamental strategy is transmitted to each of its 'gears': the decision-makers, those in charge of society.

The first gear is the consumption industry. This industry in turn determines the movements of the politicians, economists, financiers, advertisers, media, workers, retirees, unions and even the unemployed who receive support.

Inevitably, this great machine turns at the expense of human beings. It creates a way of life that seems extraordinarily rich and stimulating but is artificial and cold.

It replaces full and profound natural satisfactions with artificial ones that are superficial and ephemeral. Consumers must be constantly surprised, ever more frequently and intensely, in order to remain interested. As our civilisation speeds ever forward, constant innovation is necessary to maintain the stimulating thrill of tearing into a new package.

As the gears turn, the individual follows the movement of the group, and eventually encounters a serious problem. The ever-new satisfactions we derive from consumption, satisfactions that attract and fascinate us, are very real, and they deliver immediate pleasure. But these satisfactions are not recognised by the human reward centre, a structure that was programmed at a time when these satisfactions didn't exist. The satisfactions based on consumption are therefore unable to produce dopamine and serotonin, the chemicals that fuel our love of life.

When low levels of serotonin persist or worsen – along with the lust for life, as a consequence – we are at risk of falling below the minimum limits of satisfaction. This is the realm of unhappiness and depression.

We seek to alleviate this latent suffering, almost automatically, through the only two natural needs approved by the consumer society. The satisfaction of these needs is instantaneous and easily available: we get it from eating food and looking at screens. Too much food rich in invasive carbohydrates and too much time spent motionless in front of screens leads to weight gain, which propels the weight crisis forward. This shift is all the more hard to control since almost no one in the consumer society seems to want to fight against it.

Let's recap. The Social Pulsar emits energy, which drives the consumption industry and sustains ways of maintaining control. The consumer, targeted and enslaved, obediently consumes. The loop is closed: the consumption returns energy to the Social Pulsar, recharging its energy. This cycle explains why developed societies have increased their growth each year since the fifties, and how the weight crisis has steadily increased as a result.

The individual and society could continue to function together in this way, with great efficiency. But, at a certain point, a fundamental break between them is possible – and it's crucial to remember this point as we move forward.

It arises from the fact that each of us essentially has two minds: an ancient mind and a new mind. The new mind produces and manages consciousness, culture, technology and progress. Indeed, this is the mind that first envisioned and designed the new world of consumption. The ancient mind manages the functioning of the body, the emotions, pleasure and, above all, *survival.* Our survival absolutely depends on the love of life, instilled through the secretion of serotonin and dopamine, which is regulated by the reward circuit.

Let's look at the ten fundamental needs

These natural needs have been given fierce competition by the artificial needs that are based on consumption, but our ancient mind does not recognise consumption-based needs as reward-worthy. And that's the crux of the problem.

Hence the importance of recognising these ten fundamental needs. They have been left by the wayside; now it's time to take them back.

The ten pillars of happiness

As I have said, I developed this theory over the course of my professional life. Most of my patients who come to me because they want to lose weight tell me about the suffering they endure because of that weight. But they continue to eat in a way that can only prolong the problem.

Without their realising it, these men and women clearly eat as they do to alleviate suffering experienced by their ancient mind – in other words, suffering they experience unconsciously.

Animal observation has shown us that, when animals face stress, suffering or a threat, they try to make it stop or they flee to escape it. When fight or flight isn't an option, they opt for a third solution: they try to obtain pleasure in order to neutralise the displeasure.

Psychologists have tried to explain weight problems by looking at individual vulnerability related to childhood and early trauma. This argument is perfectly valid when it comes to explaining any given person's history. But not all of the 26 million overweight people in France – almost 7 million of whom are obese – can blame a difficult childhood. A social cause – a civilisational one, in fact – has to be at the heart of this epidemic.

When I talk to my patients who are most affected by excess weight, I *always* find suffering – not always conscious or perceived suffering, but recognisable nonetheless – vulnerability and a hypersensitivity to stress and life's challenges.

To understand the origin of this suffering, I focused on their personal histories. What I discovered was significant events or failures, often with multiple origins. Most often it was a matter of emotional difficulties, family problems and ruptured relationships. I often encountered professional problems as well, such as the inability to flourish in the workplace. Then there was a sedentary lifestyle, loss of connection with their body, isolation, spiritual emptiness, lack of self-confidence, low self-esteem, occasionally coldness, all coloured by a mood of depression.

With time and by gaining the trust of my patients, I was able to trace back the multiple origins of this suffering. In doing so, I was able to identify, one by one, those needs that, when unsatisfied, cause people to seek a substitute feeling of satisfaction through food.

The first pillar: sexuality, love and family

The first and most common of these unsatisfied needs is sexuality in the broadest sense, including love and family.

Problems within couples, divorces, estrangement from one's children, loneliness, lack of sexual relationships... Many patients who see me for weight problems or obesity have told me that their weight gain took place in a context of emotional difficulties, and that losing weight and keeping it off was much easier than dealing with these issues.

Obviously, sexuality, love and family constitute a major need. Partial or total dissatisfaction can generate profound suffering. For this reason, the sexual side of life seemed to me to be the first field of possible fulfilment, and thus the first pillar of happiness.

The second pillar: satisfaction in work and social position

The second pillar occurred to me from meeting time and again with patients who had gained a lot of weight following problems in their professional lives and difficulty succeeding in their work. Some had lost their job and were experiencing humiliation from being unemployed. I also met with patients who had been left disoriented by retirement and struggled with a sensation of uselessness and boredom. Most often, however, the men and women I spoke with found their work to be lacking joy and alienating from other humans. Nor did their job confer enough responsibility or offer room for creativity. It was simply a way to put food on the table – one that required too much travel time.

It seemed unavoidable: these complaints pointed me to the second area of fundamental need. Hence, **the second pillar**: satisfaction in work and social position.

The need to succeed in work and to reach professional heights can be so intense that it ends up obstructing other sources of satisfaction. But happiness is too meaningful and too important to be fully accessible via a single door. I've met with prominent captains of industry, people of great wealth and power, who are missing that one essential component of life.

Just as life's ups and downs have an impact on sexuality, an improvement in an individual's professional life can lead to a reduction in compulsive eating.

The third pillar: home

The third pillar was a surprise for me. In speaking to patients, I discovered the impact of *home* on patients' sense of balance and fulfilment. I noticed the importance of our need for a safe and comfortable place where we can feel at home, a space to decorate the way we want; a special place where the people we care about can come together; a place of peace and calm.

I began to realise that housing-related problems are anything but trivial. Distance from work, lack of safety, the stress of city life, the ugliness of buildings, estrangement from nature, exorbitant cost per square foot: all these have an impact on quality of life.

When the most comfortable areas of the home are centred on the refrigerator, the kitchen cupboards and the TV screen, it creates a cocktail that has powerful repercussions on weight.

But, as with the first two pillars, I believe that a change of scenery, a new location with neighbours who are friendly and welcoming to others, a place that offers some room to move, can affect how swayed we are by the attractions of shiny packaged treats. The home is a powerful thing – our equivalent to the territory that an animal will defend with its life. It is therefore the third pillar.

I'm not a psychologist, and I've never been overweight or obese. However, I was raised by women who helped me develop sensitivity and empathy. Furthermore, I take great enjoyment in being a physician. My patients are aware of that, I think; they feel comfortable telling me about their emotions, their problems and most of all their suffering.

The first time I see a patient, they will mainly talk about the suffering their excess weight causes. I've long been fascinated by the vast gap between the objective excess weight a patient has and the subjective repercussions it has on them.

After time and experience dealing with the mechanisms involved, I was able to identify a different kind of pain in the background, one that existed long before the excess weight. This original pain is in fact the cause of their eating habits and their weight problem.

What my patients tell me could be boiled down to the following: 'I'm suffering, and I eat to mask the pain and negativity with pleasure and positivity. That's how I'm able to keep going.'

But if losing weight effectively wipes out the pain linked with weight gain, the question arises: what is that original pain, the one that starts the cycle? And is there a common denominator among these diverse individual experiences of pain?

Because the global epidemic of weight problems appeared at the same time as the consumption society, it has been difficult not to interpret the weight crisis as a consequence of a lifestyle that is directly opposed to the messages carried in our genes – a lifestyle that's so very far removed from our nature.

All evidence shows that this distance from our nature damages us. It pushes those who suffer from it to find relief in other natural sources of satisfaction. For those who come to see me, the relief is in food. As a doctor and a nutritionist, I've had the opportunity to witness these patients' reality in a very personal way. Their trust in me and our emotional bond allowed me to pursue this research into these fundamental needs.

I knew that food is a vital need for the individual. I knew that sexual and familial relationships are essential for the entire species. I knew that social and professional position play a major role in self-fulfilment and self-esteem. And I knew that living in a safe and comfortable place constitutes a need as well.

I had found *three pillars*. From there my investigation continued, with great intensity: I knew that this research would reach beyond the bounds of mere nutrition. It would become a project aimed at seeing humankind's reasons for living, through a new lens.

The fourth pillar: the need for play

One constant in my life has been a keen interest in primitive man and ethology, the study of animal behaviour. Throughout my career, I've explored the origin of human-kind, examining everything from philosophy to medicine.

As a young student, I had the boldness to end up working with the zoologist and future Nobel Prize winner Konrad Lorenz. I was fascinated by this legendary man, who was famous for his unique skill as a 'goose whisperer'. Reading his work taught me that the vast majority of social animals are equipped with a *need to play*.

Lorenz saw in animal play the foundation for group bonds; he also believed it was a source of joy and a way to facilitate the ability to learn. It's clear to anyone who watches young lion cubs at play that the young animals are actually forming relationships. It's also clear that their tentative use of claws and fangs are a way to acquire, at a very young age, the gestures and postures they will use in combat: they are learning to kill. The need for play seemed so universal that it must have a crucial function.

In tandem with my medical studies, I was very inspired by anthropology courses taught by Leroy Gouran and the ethnology courses taught by Claude Lévi-Strauss. Both men helped me discover that early humans carried the raw core of humanity within them, and that understanding our ancestors would help us to learn about our own deepest needs.

The work of ethnologists and anthropologists confirmed that the animal need to play reached its culmination in humankind.

Among the Inuit, nights are spent in igloos, with everyone gathered around the fire for hours on end. The time is spent playing, miming, teasing and telling jokes. 'We tell the same stories to make everyone laugh every night: the story of a cousin who slipped on the ice, or who let the best seal of the year get away.'

Based on what my patients shared with me, this need to play was another aspect of life that seemed to be languishing. We all know that we are compelled by play, but the consumerist model tirelessly trivialises any activity that is simple and doesn't have a price tag, because they have no apparent *use*: children's games of hopscotch, card games or old-fashioned dance parties, where everyone dances together.

Our great desire for play has largely been overtaken by the passive and solitary spectacle of screens that display television shows and electronic games – which don't really form, teach or fulfil anyone.

The lack of play occurring face-to-face with other people leads to frustration. This may be less obvious than the frustration related to sex or food. But play, laughter and joy distract us. They create intervals suspended from other parts of our life. These intervals offer the chance to let anxiety and daily stresses fade. For the seventeenth-century philosopher, Pascal, recreation is one of the best strategies evolution has given us to allow us to forget – at least for a while – that life comes to an end: 'a king without diversion is a man sunk into wretchedness.' As I've often found, a similar fact is true for my patients: boredom causes hunger.

The fifth pillar: belonging to a group

Once again, it was primitive man and the great apes that pointed me towards this need, which has been drowned by the human sea of today's mega-societies.

Again, it must be understood that, for a need to enter into a species' genetic code, it must have shown that it aids the survival of the species and of its members.

Such is the case with the need to belong to a group, a need that all social animals display. Interestingly, each group has a critical mass according to species. The optimal number depends on various characteristics: anatomy, living territory, nutritional needs. A pack of bloodthirsty wolves is better equipped when hunting as a large group; a group of gorillas whose only aim is to eat tasty bamboo can be small in number, since their size makes them invulnerable. But, whatever their size and number, all social animals feel the need to belong to a group.

Jane Goodall, who spent a great deal of time among chimpanzees, found that for these animals the need is absolutely vital. Any chimpanzee rejected from its group is doomed to die. Death will occur physically, at the teeth of a predator, but also emotionally, from the trauma of being excluded from its group – like a cell or an organ separated from a body.

Of all these animals, however, humans have the strongest need for a group. Humans lack claws and fangs that provide defence or the ability to hunt. Ever since we left the trees and abandoned a fruit-based diet, we have survived, for millions of years, through cooperation within a group. This shows how the need for a group is both all-powerful and amply compensated.

But this need for a collective, to unite with others, is undermined by the gigantic size of today's societies: the number of unknown people, the disappearance of the familiar, urban life, fear and a culture of individualism.

As with most human needs, our intelligence, the accumulation and transmission of our knowledge, our progress and our culture can make our animal need for human groups seem obsolete.

But even if this were true – even if we no longer need groups to feed ourselves, defend ourselves or experience play – we still need to obtain the satisfaction (as limited as it may now be) that comes from being part of a group. If we don't get that satisfaction, we deprive ourselves of a reward that our brain ends up having to find in other ways. Failing to satisfy this need means we deprive ourselves of the intense pleasure of connection and familiarity and the extra serotonin and dopamine that nourish the desire to live.

Fortunately, there are those who find a heightened level of fulfilment and self-expression in the group, the foundation of humanity. For them, the simple and practical need for connection with others represents the opportunity to take joy in helping others. These people usually focus first and foremost on their circle of friends and family. When experience shows that it's an inexhaustible source of pleasure, they include others.

Many of my patients, however, experience this sense of belonging in only a limited way: through the choices and slogans that create a bond among an anonymous group of consumers. Some manage to avoid alienation by affirming their humanity within associations – humanitarian, charitable, environmental or political – that offer a path to fulfilment.

But others who fail to find such means are deprived of a powerful source of satisfaction. Those who lack it may unconsciously turn to other sources of natural satisfaction – the most simple and powerful of which is food.

The sixth pillar: using the body

It's the need that is most obvious of all, but also, surprisingly, the least understood and attended to. I discovered this powerful need by reading *Spark*, a book written by John J. Ratey, an American psychiatrist who undertook a thorough study of the relationship between physical and mental activity.

Ratey is one of a number of researchers who have shown the public and the medical community the extent of the organic links between physical activity and depression, stress management, hyperactivity and anxiety disorders.

It's an oft-repeated fact that physical activity is 'good for your health', one that's taken as self-evident. In fact, it's more than good for you: it's indispensable, and not just for the reasons that are usually mentioned.

To understand the essence of the need for physical

activity and the reasons for that need, you need to look deeper. Animals are different from plants since they have neither roots nor leaves, and must move around to find food and reproduce. For this activity to be effective, animals need a brain to direct and guide them.

Neuroscientists who have worked in this field have discovered, and recently proved, that physical activity in humans and animals leads to the release of serotonin. This is shown by studies conducted with groups of patients suffering from severe depression. These studies compared the effects of Zoloft, a popular antidepressant, with the effects of physical activity. The results showed that the two treatments were comparable in terms of efficacy.

Nowadays this is a well-known fact for most doctors, but the majority of people are still convinced that physical activity is only good for burning calories and to fight obesity.

But what's much less well-known, and what fascinates neuroscientists today, is that physical activity releases not just serotonin but also brain-derived neurotrophic factor (BDNF). BDNF is a growth factor that protects neurons by slowing their decline; it therefore protects memory.

But there's more – a lot more. One of the most firmly rooted dogmas of twentieth-century neurology is that we come into the world with a limited number of neurons, and that, starting from the end of early childhood, we lose them each day, with no hope of getting more. In 1998, however, this dogma was shattered by the chance discovery that certain parts of the brain could create new nerve cells from stem cells.

This neuronal regeneration is controlled by BDNF, and physical activity stimulates its release. This represents a great hope for the possibility of delaying or mitigating degenerative brain diseases such as Alzheimer's or Parkinson's.

But at another level, seemingly far removed from the topic of serious diseases, consider that only thirty minutes of jogging or one hour of walking per day improves not only your mood but also your intellectual power.

For all these reasons, engaging your body is one of the fundamental needs whose satisfaction offers a wealth of fulfilment. It's part of the formula for happiness. Yet the majority of patients who come to see me for obesity, excess weight or diabetes are extremely sedentary. A sedentary lifestyle is an inherent part of our way of life today: one out of two patents filed today is intended to save time or reduce physical activity.

Our widespread and pervasive dependence on effort-saving machines implies that modernity and technological progress have made physical activity a thing of the past, relegating it to the status of merely a task or chore. Certainly, as we see on a daily basis, it may be possible to survive with an extremely low level of activity. But doing so deprives us of a proven, undeniable source of satisfaction.

The seventh pillar: experience nature

The seventh pillar is another simple and obvious need, so much so that it took me some time to discover it. It's nothing more than the need to experience nature. It's superfluous to say that we humans need nature: we ourselves are an element of nature. There's no need to wax philosophical or moral to explain it. Brain imaging has shown that immersion in nature, walking in the forest or near the ocean, near plants and animals, activates the reward centres in the brain.

Our distance from this miraculous cradle of life comes from the fact that we've come to think that urban life has more value and utility than nature. Nature just doesn't provide the same bombardment of visual and auditory stimulation.[6]

And yet, once again, there's a vast difference between what culture tells us and what nature shows us. Trees, flowers, leaves, forests, smells, colours, the sky and the clouds, wind and storms, the ocean with its waves and their salty spray, the soil, sand, rivers, wild animals: they fascinate us because we are programmed to hear them, see them and inhale them. Each moment nature calls to us, every message it emits to us, is recognised by

---

[6] In 1960, 33.6 per cent of the world's population was living in urban areas; in 2014 the percentage had risen to 53.4 per cent. Source: World Bank (http://databank.banquemondiale.org/data/reports). In 2012, the OECD estimated that 70 per cent of the world's population will be urban by 2050 (http://www.oecd.org/fr/env/indicateurs-modelisation-perspectives/49884240.pdf).

our ancient mind, our instinctual side, as a sign that we belong and are connected to *life*. And each moment we connect with nature is rewarded, giving us reassurance and helping us live.

When I realised this, it was clear that I had found my seventh need.

So how do we connect with nature today? René Char, a renowned French poet and philosopher, wrote to me one day with an observation: 'Forests are sleeping within our gardens.' For most of us, gardens have become a luxury. But something as simple as a potted geranium on a balcony, with care given to its leaves and to its general presentation, shows that the link is not totally broken.

Pets are another outlet for our need for nature. And there are others: an overcrowded beach that's nonetheless a small sanctuary for nature, a children's park or a garden, spots for hunting or fishing, horseback riding for those who have the luxury, even hobby farms and animal husbandry.

But all these things share a single disadvantage: they are free. That means there's no incentive for businesses to let us enjoy our happiness. How can we be happy when we reject our natural environment, our origin and our status as animals? Humans have reached a unique state of self-consciousness, but that doesn't make us extra-terrestrials. On the contrary: that consciousness, and the scientific knowledge that has emerged from it, has found the proof that experiencing nature is a simple way to create satisfaction and the desire to live.

But there's reason to have hope. This need can easily be brought back to the forefront of our lives; it can even be boosted by combining it with physical activity. It's easy to run or walk in a forest or barefoot on the sand, or to bring a domesticated animal into your life: the horses we ride, the dogs that protect our homes and the cats that offer warmth and affection.

The eighth and ninth pillars: unique to humans

You may have noticed that all the needs we've looked at thus far are shared by humans and animals alike. Like us, animals need to eat food, reproduce, move freely in an environment they feel a part of, live as a meaningful part of a group and feel safe within its territory.

Now let's look at the two needs that belong to humans alone: the need for spirituality, and the need for beauty.

The eighth pillar: spirituality and transcendence

The need for spirituality is unique to humans. But it was also present in the form of man that preceded us: the Neanderthals. We know that Neanderthals buried their dead, and decorated the departed, placing at their side objects that they loved while living. For prehistorians, this fact alone proves that these creatures had a sense of the sacred. Their approach to burial shows that the Neanderthals had a spirituality that rejected death; they saw it instead as merely the passage to another life.

No matter how far back we look, there is no group,

society or civilisation in our species that has lived without bending a knee and looking towards the heavens. Each has expressed it in its own way: totems, magic, ancestor worship, fascination with natural forces, petitions to gods, search for superhuman powers, the search for the absolute, violent rites and myths.

Why is this urge so ubiquitous in humans?

Between the last of the apes and the first humans, a crucial event took place: the appearance of self-consciousness. This is not the basic consciousness involved in existing and acting, which other higher animals possess, but something else: the consciousness of being conscious. The event is unprecedented in the evolution of life, and it opened the door to a terrifying reality. Man discovered that his death was inevitable. This revelation represented an unimaginable threat to this new and fragile species. How could people live each day with the certitude that they would one day die?

Pascal wrote a famous meditation on the fear of death. 'Imagine a number of men in chains, all under sentence of death, some of whom are each day butchered in the sight of the others; those remaining see their own condition in that of their fellows, and looking at each other with grief and despair await their turn. This is an image of the human condition.'

But, as always, evolution chose life: it found a way to protect our promising species. From the first humans with self-consciousness, it selected for survival those whose brains were well suited to contemplate the irrational and the invisible. This would open up a way to neutralise the terrifying anxiety of our inevitable end.

This is probably how the drive towards the sacred ended up being written into our DNA. Contemplating the spiritual became a way of protecting life. We know that prayer, meditation and faith produce serotonin and dopamine. The need to believe in something bigger than ourselves helps us to live. That's why a sense of the sacred crossed all cultures, eras and territories, without exception.

For the first time since our origins, however, that need for the sacred has crumbled under the assault of progress, science and technology – in just a few generations. For a great many, spirituality has all but disappeared. The new idols of consumption have taken the place of the divine.

But the actual need remains undeniable, and offers an incredible source of power for achieving peace – for some, even seemingly heavenly joy. The eighth pillar is therefore spirituality and the sacred.

The ninth pillar (and the newest arrival): beauty, wonder, the aesthetic experience

How can we explain this need, which no animal seems to experience? What's the reason for the appearance of this intangible attribute, which in a way seems so useless? What good does beauty really do? Why is beauty, like the sacred, written into our programming?

The answer is tied to the previous pillar. The need for

the sacred entered our programming when humans were compelled to address the invisible. But our daily language, as profane as it is, was simply inadequate to establish some connection with a god or creator. It seemed inappropriate, even disrespectful.

Thus, to separate ourselves from the profane, another language was born: the language of art. There were the fantastic cave markings, such as at Lascaux and Altamira, totems, sacred masks, carvings, sculptures, religious music, hieroglyphics, temple decorations, churches, cathedrals and altarpieces. Art is the manifestation of the beautiful. Although the creation of art is the prerogative of artists, the aesthetic feeling it produces belongs to every human. That's why for most of history, art has almost always been both religious and anonymous.

It was during the Italian Renaissance that art became secularised, detached from religion; that's when artists first started signing their works. With this gesture, they entered into what would later be called the art market. These were the first hints of consumer society beginning to see the beautiful as merchandise, when previously it was more concerned with utility. It would also give rise to extravagance, scandal and provocation as a part of the world of art. Marcel Duchamp probably marked the height of this shift, when he exhibited in a museum an upside-down shop-bought porcelain urinal, which he signed and titled 'Fountain'.

Once again, the same forces are at play. They aim to

distract us from natural, free sources of satisfaction and to replace them with those that support the economy.

The beautiful is not beautiful in and of itself. We find things beautiful because our brain has been programmed to recognise signals of beauty and then to create reward. The process is the same as with the eight other needs we've looked at. On the surface, aesthetic emotion generates an intense feeling of pleasure. But, on a deeper level, it stimulates a discharge of serotonin and dopamine, which recharges the will to live. The need for beauty is the ninth pillar of happiness.

The tenth pillar: food

The tenth pillar in my theory is the one that's at the heart of this project. It's the category of food, oral consumption, what you put in your mouth.

Without this constant and powerful impulse, life wouldn't last more than a few weeks. This need involves powerful pleasures and high levels of rewards.

And it's here that consumer culture has found its golden goose. Food is the ultimate human need, the subject of a vital and fundamental drive that can be exploited and commercialised to the fullest extent. Thus, the consumption industry's strategy is the exact opposite of its strategy for other needs. While it usually works by imposing restrictions, for food it opts for exponential increase. This is done through industrial processing to make products more concentrated, and by carefully honing the sensory message attached to products. These all combine to make modern food products as addictive as possible.

There's another human need that has similarly been co-opted and bound to its economic function: recreation. The need for food and the need for play both now revolve around addiction and profit. Play takes place via various glowing screens: television, with its explosion of channels; electronic games that are ever-more invasive and addictive; and the Internet and its related devices, which are probably just in their infancy.

I'm well suited to be your guide into the workings of this mechanism because I witnessed its birth – I was born around the same time as the weight crisis – and I have observed it at length in my practice as a medical nutritionist. So now let's summarise this long development simply and clearly.

Entering into the role of consumer has deeply changed how we live. Population pressures and the goal of indefinite growth, propelled by constant technological advances, have locked us into the status of consumers. To solidify this status, every effort has been made to diminish natural satisfactions, the pleasures that are immediate and free, to replace them with profitable ones in the form of food and games.

This new equation, which runs counter to human nature and the natural world, creates suffering. This suffering automatically seeks alleviation. We grasp on to anything we can obtain in shops, seeking the satisfaction provided by food and screens.

The reduced scope of our satisfactions leaves us in a compulsive state, and results in a constant state of demand. It pushes us to eat too much and badly, and to remain sedentary. That's the basic explanation for how we have become machines for producing excess weight, obesity and diabetes, in just two generations.

Now when I speak with a new patient who has problems with excess weight and diabetes, I ask a number of questions systematically to explore each of the natural sources of fulfilment. Almost every time, I see that their weight gain has developed in parallel with a decrease in happiness in many of these areas.

The more areas lacking satisfaction, the more desperate and inescapable our compulsion to eat and our willingness to avoid movement by finding distraction in front of a screen.

If a woman tells me that she is widowed or divorced and that her children or grandchildren live far away, there's a good chance she's not finding satisfaction in love, sexuality and family.

If she is retired, unemployed or doesn't enjoy her work, she is cut off from the second field of fulfilment.

If she doesn't like where she lives, another door is closed.

If she has an urban lifestyle and lacks connection with nature, yet another door shuts.

And, if she has ended up in a somewhat solitary life and is sometimes marginalised because she is overweight, she may find herself without a community.

Finally, if the spiritual and aesthetic side of life is absent, everything seems to lead to a choice between two terrible options: depression or obesity.

I don't think I've ever seen anyone who has deficiencies in all of these areas combined. But among those who have gained a lot of weight over a long period of time, I have observed less success in obtaining the simple, natural and basic satisfactions.

My next book, which will be titled *The Ten Pillars of Happiness*, will explain this fundamental process that, for the first time in human history, has enslaved the individual and compromised their happiness for the benefit of society. My position as author is not limited to that of observer and analyst, however. This book will also be a source of new ideas on how to understand and reverse the trend.

We know that physical activity is capable of inducing dopamine and serotonin secretion. Walking twenty minutes each day can produce enough of these chemicals to silence the demand for foods eaten merely for gratification.

Just as it's possible to use physical activity to lessen the need to put food in your mouth, it's possible – or well worth trying, at least – to do the same in other areas you've been neglecting. It could be by playing a musical instrument, reading life-changing books, reconnecting with nature, meeting new people and enjoying sexuality, or adopting a lovable pet.

But it all starts with diagnosing the problem.

CHAPTER 4

Sugars and the Lobbies that Promote Them

The public finally started hearing warnings about the dangers of sugars in the seventies. The warnings were prompted by scientists who were concerned about the exaggeration and misinformation they saw in the war against fat and cholesterol in the United States. Ostensibly, this war had started because of the role of fat and cholesterol in the incidence of cardiovascular disease. And, almost automatically, restriction of fats opened the door wide for the broad carbohydrate family, which includes all sugars.

The attack on fat and cholesterol, which began in the United States and was spread throughout the media, largely started with Ancel Keys, an ambitious professor at the University of Minnesota. Keys made his reputation with the Seven Countries Study, which he led in 1956. The study showed that countries such as Finland and the

United States that consumed large amounts of animal fats also had high rates of heart attack. Countries in southern Europe, however, such as Greece or Italy, that consumed more carbohydrates and vegetable fats had lower heart attack rates.

It was on this shaky premise that the fierce crusade against cholesterol and high-fat foods began. And in order to fill the significant dent that this made in the human diet, a blank cheque was written for the consumption of carbohydrate-heavy foods. Moreover, this occurred at a crucial moment, when the food industry started gaining access to high technology for processing and refining carbohydrates.

Today we know that that study was biased. The seven countries had been deliberately selected to get the hoped-for results. Thus, France, the land of cheese, steak and mayonnaise, was cast aside, because its heart attack rate was relatively low. Inversely, Chile was ignored since its heart attack rate was high but its fat consumption was low.

Furthermore, in recent years, many have been asking how a movement of such magnitude could have begun and spread around the world over half a century, when its scientific foundation was so questionable – and when its claims had such far-reaching consequences. Many point to the power of the lobbies for the sugar and pharmaceutical industry; the former profits directly from the sugar industry, and the second profits from diseases that result from sugar consumption.

But whatever the reason, at the time this study – which had such a massive impact on the public – was supported and promoted by the media, politicians and scientific authorities. The majority of America's nutritionists followed suit.

In 1961, Keys received the support of the American Heart Association, the country's leading scientific body. Their endorsement gave him unshakeable authority and earned him the nickname 'Mr Cholesterol'.

Things went so far during that time that shoppers were offered blood tests for cholesterol in supermarkets in the United States.

It was in 1972, in the midst of this fervour, that a book was published by John Yudkin, professor of nutrition at the University of London.

This book, which came from a recognised authority, created a scandal: it directly contradicted Keys' position.

Yudkin said that fats were not to blame; sugar was primarily responsible for heart disease.

The sugar lobby got involved, contradicting his carefully developed theory. Yudkin was forced to use every tool he had to stand up to what he saw as a threat to his integrity. He was opposing an industry that until that time had exercised its power without meeting any resistance.

Yudkin was personally attacked and portrayed as a fanatic; his ideas were dismissed as 'emotional assertions'. As a result of the media lynching, he was discredited and marginalised by the scientific community. He found himself unable to publish. As all this was transpiring, the sugar industry was funding studies to show that sugars are benign, bolstering their claim with relentless advertising and the creation of ever more addictive and seductive products.[7]

When Yudkin died in 1995, he was defeated and forgotten.

In 1972, cardiologist Robert Atkins entered the fray, publishing *Dr. Atkins' New Diet Revolution*, a book that became an international bestseller. His weight-loss method differed from Keys' in every way. It was based on drastic reduction of all carbohydrates, and removed all limits on fats. After an intense wave of success, Atkins became subject to attacks as virulent as those Yudkin had faced.

Twenty years later, many doctors and nutritionists recognised that Atkins had been correct. Walter Willett, head of the world's leading nutrition research centre, Harvard School of Public Health, believes that Atkins was unfairly targeted.

In 1980, Professor David Jenkins created and began promoting the concept of the glycaemic index, which would become a major tool in the prevention of diabetes and weight problems. This index measures food absorption and the impact of that absorption on blood glucose concentrations and insulin secretion. The major advantage of this index is that it used provable facts and

---

[7] Sacks, F.M., Bray, G.A., Carey, V.J. et al., 'Comparison of weight-loss diets with different compositions of fat, protein and carbohydrates', *The New England Journal of Medicine*, 2009, 360 (9), p 859-873

numbers to show the degree of toxicity of a carbohydrate-containing food.

By insisting that sugar is one of the most penetrating carbohydrates – and therefore one of the most dangerous – Jenkins too came under heavy fire, drawing criticism and unconcealed hostility from lobbies. Today he says, 'I see myself as someone who has always been under the heat of controversy because the concepts I introduced were new to their times.'[8]

Today, the glycaemic index concept is an undeniable scientific fact. It gives us a simple way to show the impact of different foods on the pancreas. Now that the entire international community is deeply concerned with the weight and diabetes epidemic and wants to find a solution, the nutritional labels on food packaging are poised to be the primary tool to protect consumers and the public. But this labelling, which brings down the sugar industry and even more so the flour industry, is not permitted today. In my view, this restriction is absolutely a health scandal. I have been pushing to make this labelling mandatory for years now.

Picture yourself shopping in a supermarket. As you walk down the aisle, you decide to bring a smile to the face of your young child, and you grab a box of corn flakes from the shelf. Television commercials have told you that the cereal,

[8] Source: www.lanutrition.fr (www.lanutrition.fr/bien-comprendre/le-potential-sante-des-aliments/index-et-charge-glycemiques/pr-david-jenkins-les-sedentaires-beneficient-du-regime-ig)

served with milk, is an ideal healthy meal for your child. But, as you're about to put the colourful box into your cart, something catches your eye: a bright-red warning showing the cereal's glycaemic index level. You take a closer look. The glycaemic index is 80 – higher than white sugar.

Today, however, this labelling, which would do so much to protect the consumer is prohibited. It's nothing short of an outrage.

Basing his work on Jenkins' discoveries, Michel Montignac made waves in the nineties by offering a new weight-loss method. Like Jenkins, Montignac recommended excluding sugars – and, by extension, the carbohydrates with the highest glycaemic indexes – from one's diet. And, like Jenkins, Montignac faced fierce attacks from lobbies, which used the fact that he wasn't a doctor as extra ammunition.

The lobbies for the sugar and white flour industries wield enormous hidden power on our political decision-makers, the media and advertising agencies, the medical community and the general public.

The smear campaigns mentioned above aren't their only tactic: these lobbies have mastered a carefully constructed strategy of misinformation. The strategy boils down to this: create maximum promotion for sugary and floury products, and put out effective counter-advertising for any and all who point out the dangers.

One of their most effective methods is to try to draw our attention away from the only weapon we have to fight obesity and diabetes: diet. The mouthpieces for this attack are often psychologists. For them, diet is something of an easy target; they may talk about the unbearable trauma that a diet can bring. It also comes from certain doctors, from consultants who are getting paid by the biggest brands in the sugar industry, from associations looking for sponsors, from researchers angling to receive funding.

But we also see another approach: ineffective diets are endorsed, while truly effective diets – which represent a financial threat – are criticised. The most glaring example of this is that we continue to see diets based on calorie counting, even after fifty years of failure. The only explanation for the continued popularity of these diets, which we are finally realising are counterproductive, is that lobbies have persistently supported them.

The calorie-based concept of diet is actually based on a dogmatic assertion: **'All calories are equal, regardless of their origin'.**

Every doctor knows that this claim is false. But repeated often enough, a mistruth becomes accepted as fact.

For fifty years, it has been held as true – against the evidence – that 100 calories from fish is equal to 100 calories from sugar. Why did the doctors who supported that view ignore the fact that diabetes develops because of sugar's toxicity, and not because of calories? Why did they overlook the fact that 80 per cent of diabetics are overweight, and that insulin controls sugar by turning it into fat?

But today, the dogma of calories, which paralysed the

fight against invasive sugars and the weight crisis, is finally starting to be discredited. Health authorities are being forced to take responsibility, and, facing pressure from the World Health Organization (WHO), are starting to change their position. But unfortunately this change doesn't equal victory: the calorie dogma is being replaced with an ever more insidious view. Since the calorie dogma is untenable, our attention is being drawn away from diets altogether. The message: Diets are useless.

Hence, a leading voice in the US launched a campaign, which has become ubiquitous in France: Stop Dieting. Commentators with no medical training rushed to support the trend. Coaches, bloggers, and more, all claimed to have lost dozens of kilograms without having given up any foods.

Then there's the argument put forward by various psychologists who have suggested that watching your diet is equivalent to abuse, a kind of 'cognitive restriction'. Some have even described dieting as 'orthorexia nervosa', a condition that can lead to severe consequences for mental health. These voices tell us that all you need to do to lose weight is 'listen to your feelings', to make a distinction between craving and hunger – or, better still, to simply accept your weight.

When you need to lose weight but you lack the necessary motivation, it's comforting to hear that dieting only leads to frustration and to unpreventable binge-eating that is actually the sole cause of the weight and obesity crisis. Lobbies have so much power that they can tell the world – without fear of ridicule – that 2 billion overweight people and half a billion diabetics are *victims of their own attempts to lose weight.* And then there's the 20 per cent of people who have lost weight and still haven't regained it five years later – a group that this view conveniently fails to account for.

An even more sophisticated stratagem emerged a few years ago: the concept of **balance**. To lose weight, all you need to do is have a balanced diet: a bit of everything, but in moderation.

Who could oppose a concept as noble and pure as *balance?* However, those who have helped obese people lose weight and who know what these people go through are aware that we don't gain weight by choosing the wrong foods; we get bigger because we make choices that are rooted in our pain, and *ignore* whether the foods are fattening. The word 'compulsive' is the key here. Those who are prone to compulsive behaviour suffer from being overweight; but they suffer even more if they deny themselves the foods that cause weight gain.

Eating in a balanced way is healthy and worthwhile. Such a diet no doubt makes it possible to stabilise your weight; but it in no way helps you *lose* weight. As a solution for obese people, it's simply not the answer.

For five years now, the leading voices in the scientific community in the United States – the country with the highest obesity and diabetes rates – have been warning us about the dangers of sugar.

One of these voices belongs to Robert Lustig, professor of paediatric endocrinology at the University of California. Lustig has probably done more work than anyone else today on sugar and fructose. He considers them poisons: 'Sugar,' he said, 'is the biggest culprit of the country's explosive rate of obesity. Sugar has poisoned food and disrupted people's biology.'[9]

Lobbies continue to oppose Lustig's claims and struggle to reduce the impact of his work. But it's becoming harder for them to hide the seriousness of the health epidemic in the United States, or the soaring numbers of child and adolescent diabetes. Lustig's reputation, his position in the scientific community, and his charisma and ability to inspire trust has given him a degree of immunity that Yudkin, Atkins and Montignac lacked. In a country where lobbies have a staggering amount of power, Lustig has the courage to tell us, 'the food industry has its hands free to put any amount of sugar in any food it wants. That is the problem.'

Lustig is aiming at more than just obesity and diabetes. He considers these to be elements of the broader issue of metabolic syndrome. His focus as a paediatrician is on the tragic effects of our modern-day diet on human beings at an extremely young age. In his view, sugar and fructose are 'alcohol for children'; in the same way that alcohol can destroy an alcoholic's cirrhotic liver, sugar is capable of profoundly altering the liver's functioning and structure.

---

[9] Watch his talk online at www.youtube.com/watch?v=dBnniua6

SUGARS AND THE LOBBIES THAT PROMOTE THEM

Metabolic syndrome is affecting growing numbers of children today. It now includes excess abdominal weight (belly fat), hypertension, high cholesterol, high triglycerides, fatty liver and diabetes. And Lustig predicts that, when today's children reach adulthood, they will face frighteningly widespread levels of heart attacks.

Very recently, he conducted a study on the effects of hidden sugars on this metabolic disorder, which is affecting children in such large numbers.

For this study, his team selected obese children who consumed too much added sugar and fructose and who had high blood pressure, high fasting blood glucose levels, high insulin levels and elevated liver enzymes, along with obesity.

The diet developed for these children reduced or replaced sugars from fruits, grains, bread and pasta, **but without changing the number of calories taken in by the children.**

After only nine days of this diet, the benefits were remarkable. All the parameters improved, without any weight loss whatsoever. Blood pressure dropped, blood glucose and insulin levels dropped, triglycerides plummeted, bad cholesterol dropped, good cholesterol rose and the liver reduced in size, and their biological markers improved.

What this study confirms is that all calories are *not* equal, and that only those with 'added sugars' are responsible for metabolic disorders leading to diabetes, obesity and fatty liver.

The subject is complex, but Lustig's demonstration is

shockingly clear. I strongly recommend watching *Sugar: The Bitter Truth*, a documentary that has received 6 million views on YouTube since it was released in 2009. **The lesson of the documentary can be summed up in five words: Beware of sugar and fructose.**

As a paediatrician, Lustig believes that the younger the child, the more dangerous their exposure to sugar and fructose, and the greater the necessity for prevention. Lustig and I are allies in this respect, and on the whole, I support his message and his project.

In 1969, I wrote the first book about a diet that would end up being named after me. This diet was founded, theoretically, on the elimination of sugars. Today, I aim to go further, by tackling the problem at the root. That means asking pregnant women to limit – for the most susceptible months of pregnancy – exposure to sugars of the foetus that will be brought into the world.

CHAPTER 5

The Engine that Drives the Weight Crisis: Insulin and the Pancreas

Chapter 2 was meant to draw your attention to the dangers and consequences that are directly linked with excess weight. The idea was to make you aware that there is in fact a powerful solution – *and that the solution is in your own hands.*

In Chapters 3 and 4, we looked at the emotional, mental and social components of the weight crisis. Our focus was on the awe-inspiring power created by the balance that exists between supply and demand.

Now, in this chapter, I will present the main actor in the weight and diabetes crisis: the pancreas.

As I have explained, this book is aimed at a generation of women who are learning how to bring the next generation into being. As you prepare to create new life, you will simultaneously be targeted by a diet that has become increasingly artificial over the last thirty years, and that contains far too many processed carbohydrates. This new diet may be tolerable for adult women in the medium term – but the same isn't true for a developing foetus.

Indeed, in just thirty years, our modern diet has resulted in two generations of newborns that are born larger than previous generations, and that are afflicted with a *latent vulnerability*. This vulnerability is the cause for a two-pronged crisis: excess weight and diabetes.

That's my theory; now it has to be proven. The key piece of evidence is the pancreas – your own pancreas (and it's important to understand how it works), but especially the pancreas of your unborn child, which is absolutely more sensitive and vulnerable than your own.

An adult pancreas has many functions. What we're most concerned with here is its function as an endocrine gland: the pancreas secretes insulin, among other things. Insulin is a hormone that plays an important role in human physiology. One of its main purposes is to regulate a person's blood glucose level (ideally, in the context of a natural human diet). After each meal containing carbohydrates, the pancreas prevents concentrations of glucose in your blood from reaching levels that would be extremely toxic for all the organs that the blood reaches.

Today, however, the human pancreas is forced to behave differently than in the past. That's because it is responding to the invasion of foods that *did not exist* at the time when the pancreas was 'programmed'. If you have a cat or dog, you've probably been told by a veterinarian at some point that you shouldn't feed it sugar.

This chapter is not meant for those who already have some knowledge of the science; they probably know the facts already. It's meant for you: a mother-to-be who doesn't want her child to be at risk, to be yet another sufferer of the plague that now strikes just over one out of every two adults.[10]

The window for establishing protection against the new foods that have flooded our diet comes at the end of your third month of pregnancy. That's when the first cells of your foetus's pancreas start preparing to secrete insulin.

I've said it before, but it's worth repeating: the human pancreas has existed and secreted insulin for millions of years now – since long before bakeries even existed. Unfortunately, this self-evident fact is generally covered up or denied by those who manufacture the food products that are so high in invasive carbohydrates.

Now let's open our eyes to another simple fact. If today's diet harms and overworks the adult pancreas, the assault is infinitely more damaging for the nascent pancreas of a foetus developing in its mother's womb.

What actually happens

It's important that you follow with me step by step as we move forward. To begin, then, let's take a closer look at

---

[10] Source: IASO, 27 May 2014 (www.oecd.org/health/obesity-update)

an experience that each of us has on a daily basis. It's an experience that usually goes unexamined; but, when you break it down, it tends to cause what's known as a 'eureka moment'. Once you understand what's happening, there's no going back.

So let's proceed.

1) If you are an adult human female, you have 5 litres of blood in your body.

2) If you are not diabetic, your blood has approximately 1 gram of glucose per litre, fasting.

3) If you have between 1.10 and 1.25 grams, you are hyperreactive to sugar, and tolerate it poorly.

   If you have 1.26 grams or higher, fasting, you're considered diabetic.

4) Obviously, if a litre of blood contains 1 gram of glucose, 5 litres contains 5 grams. Based on the total volume of your blood, that equals barely more than a teaspoon of white sugar.

Now, let's imagine a typical situation. You're in a supermarket and you buy a normal packet of biscuits for you or your family. You're feeling stressed, or just rushed, so you open the packet. You put one biscuit in your mouth, then another – over the next fifteen minutes, you end up eating about a third of the packet. It's okay, you tell yourself: you aren't the first to resort to sweet treats to calm yourself down and have a little enjoyment.

Now, before you throw the packet in the bin, you stop and read the nutritional information. The first line on the rectangular label will probably tell you the number of calories per serving; a serving may be around 100 grams.

Lower down on the label, you'll find the information we're really after: the total carbohydrates, the amount of 'sugars' in a serving of the product.

If it's a typical biscuit, the amount will be between about 60 and 70 grams per 100 grams – the average would be 65 grams for an average weight of 170 grams.

So, by consuming that generous helping of biscuits, you will have ingested 110 grams of carbohydrates in the form of white flour and sugar. Carbohydrates are among the most invasive sugars; they end up in your blood within half an hour.

With the 5 grams you already had in your blood, this influx ends up raising the total blood sugar level massively: 5 grams + 110 grams = 115 grams.

At the litre level, this would bring your blood glucose level to around 23 grams per litre. Any doctor will tell you that no human can survive with a blood sugar level that high: at 10 grams per litre, you're at risk of falling into a diabetic coma.

But we know from everyday experience that, unless you have severe diabetes, you won't really die from eating a packet of biscuits.

How do we explain this apparent contradiction?

The explanation is simple. Since you're not in the final stage of diabetes, your pancreas is able to perform its basic function and control your blood sugar level. Here's what happens, in closer detail:

It all starts in the moment when you decide to buy the biscuits and open the packet. Your pancreas receives a signal and starts to anticipate what's coming by secreting insulin. Then, as the biscuits enter your mouth and start to get digested, the secretion accelerates. Finally, when the sugars enter the blood and get converted into glucose, a massive amount of insulin is released to deal with this **potentially life-threatening inundation**.

Insulin has only limited and poorly adapted means to deal with the situation. It may be starting to seem like a mantra: no pancreas, animal or human was designed to face foods that are as rich in sugar, as penetrating and invasive, as sucrose (white table sugar), *and, even worse, today's white flour.*

With no natural means of destroying this excess glucose, your body has a different way to counter the problem: flushing it out of the blood.

The sugars expelled from the blood end up being stored in three places. These physiological storage facilities are the muscle, the liver and the adipose tissue.

- The human liver is able to store 50 grams of glucose in a compressed form: glycogen. But the liver of today's sedentary human is usually dealing with a backlog of sugar. Still dealing with the sugars that accumulated during the previous meal, it can absorb only a small part of the new sugars coming in.

- The glucose therefore tries to rest in the muscles, which normally consume a lot of glucose, storing it in the form of glycogen. But the situation ends up being the same as with the liver. The muscles of the average person today are insufficiently used. They are overloaded with accumulated glycogen and can take in only a small portion of the sugar.
- And so the disturbing amounts of glucose finally head for the fatty tissue. There they encounter no obstacles. That's because the primary role of the adipose tissue (also called fatty tissue) is to store energy in the form of fat: the material designed by evolution to pack a maximum of calories into a minimum of space. Fatty tissue in a human being can easily take in a million calories.

The reality is infinitely more complex than what I've described, of course – but that, in a nutshell, is the process.

Faced with such an onslaught of this highly toxic nutrient, insulin has to adapt to a situation for which it is not prepared. It converts the heavy dose of lethal poison into a substance that's fully tolerated by the organism: fat. **It's no exaggeration to say that insulin saves your life by taking on the threat – but it does so at the cost of weight gain that makes you fat.**

Now, for those who want to know more (without getting extremely technical), here's what happens in closer detail:

To cope with the powerful and sizeable blood sugar increase, the pancreas puts a comprehensive emergency plan into action.

From the moment that you start mentally anticipating a sugary treat, secreted insulin stops the body from using free fatty acids in order to give full priority to glucose circulating in the blood.

To do so, insulin activates two antagonistic enzymes.

Stimulation of lipoprotein lipase (LPL)

LPL is an enzyme that binds fat. Its job is to capture the fats circulating in the blood and store them in any cells that will take them – fat cells, mainly. It targets small fatty acids that move easily in both directions between adipocytes and the bloodstream. Triglycerides, as their name implies, consist of three fatty acids connected by a glycerol molecule. Their large size makes them less mobile; they therefore end up being stored long term.

LPL also prevents muscles from burning fatty acids so that glycogen is used up instead.

Inhibition of hormone-sensitive lipase (HSL)

HSL is another enzyme that liberates fats. Its role is exactly the opposite of LPL's role. HSL dismantles triglyceride molecules that, because of their size, are stored in the adipose tissue. This releases fatty acids into the bloodstream, where they disperse. HSL thus effectively facilitates the burning of fats, and therefore weight loss.

Insulin, however, blocks HSL, so that glucose combustion has top priority and activates the metabolism of glucose into fat. Adipocytes absorb glucose and use up glycerol, a carbohydrate that combines with fatty acids to form triglycerides.

Finally, insulin has the ability to activate the creation of new adipose cells to further increase fat-storage ability.

Insulin thus facilitates the storage of fat in a number of ways. That means it has the effect of causing weight gain. Indeed, that's not a surprise: we've been aware of the relation between insulin and weight gain since the sixties.

The science can get complicated, but there's a simple way to frame all this. In the words of Harvard professor Georges Cahill:

'Carbohydrate is driving insulin is driving fat.'

And since insulin production is triggered by carbohydrate consumption, *carbohydrates* are primarily to blame for weight gain.

This is shown by the direct, chronological correlation between the diabesity crisis and the massive spread of processed foods, rich in invasive carbohydrates, in today's diet.

The biggest factor in the secretion of insulin is the *kind* of carbohydrate ingested. The type of carbohydrate determines how upset the pancreas will become, and how much insulin it will secrete as a result. More specifically, a carbohydrate's power to cause weight gain is determined by the ease with which it will be digested and absorbed.

Never before in human history has our species had so much access to carbohydrate-laden foods – foods that are

artificial and reconstituted like never before – as it has during the last two generations' lifetime.

When looking at the development of the three types of nutrients – proteins, fats and carbohydrates – over the last fifty years, what becomes clear?

For protein-heavy foods such as meat, fish, poultry, seafood or eggs, little has changed in terms of nutritional value. A steak, an egg or a piece of salmon wouldn't look very different today to how it did in the seventies.

The same goes for fats – olive oil and butter aren't much different today to how they were generations ago.

But it's a very different story when it comes to carbohydrates. Their production started to soar about fifty years ago. Walking through any supermarket today, you'll see that the selection of these enticing foods is endlessly growing. What's more, their composition and heightened sugar content make them truly addictive.

Sugars, insulin, long-term effects

What will happen if the dynamic between sugar, insulin and weight gain continues to progress the way it's been going since about 1965 to 1970, with fats being demonised and sugars taking their place in the diet?

Only twenty years ago, when all-out war was waged in the United States against cholesterol and fat – a war that history will show was ill advised – here's what the American Heart Association was saying:

'In order to control the amount and type of saturated

fatty acids and cholesterol you consume, choose snacks from other food groups such as lighter crackers, salt-free pretzels, sweets, sugar, syrup, honey or jam.'

Above, we looked at the one-off effects of a single packet of biscuits on an adult pancreas. But what happens if this consumption of invasive carbohydrates happens on a daily basis? What it leads to is an equally regular secretion of insulin – and therefore to increasing weight gain. And this is the situation for the great majority of people who are overweight or obese or have diabetes.

Imagine the case of an overweight person who, instead of eating meat, fish and green vegetables, regularly consumes white bread, potatoes, fruit juice, white rice from Chinese or Japanese restaurants, biscuits in the afternoon, doesn't shy away from beer and adds two teaspoons of sugar to their coffee. Then there's the next level up: those who drink sugary fizzy drinks and eat dips, crisps and sweets.

I think that many people, especially those who are experiencing weight problems, would think that this is a pretty normal diet, and would admit that it's quite similar to their own.

We've considered what happens when insulin, to safeguard against high levels of glucose in the blood, activates fat production and causes excess weight. But what happens if a diet too high in 'sugars' persists and becomes a daily occurrence?

After some time – varying from person to person and according to the amount of sugars being consumed – a phenomenon arises that is truly disastrous for the organism: *insulin resistance*. (Remember the term; it will become as crucial as the term *glycaemic index*.)

How does insulin resistance happen? The short answer: too many fast carbohydrates, and too little insulin.

Gradually, the body's cells responsible for mopping up excess glucose start to be affected by the toxicity of the sugar. Battered and exhausted, unable to do their job, these cells end up resisting the orders they receive from insulin.

To compensate for that resistance and ensure your survival, the pancreas must therefore secrete a little more insulin to obtain the same result. But over time, the resistance increases. This leads to two consequences.

As we've already seen, more insulin equals more weight gain. If the consumption of sugars continues and is not corrected – if it becomes addictive – extra weight quickly becomes obesity.

During all this, the strength or weakness of the person's pancreas becomes a factor. Over time, increased and prolonged exertion by the pancreas can end up wearing out the organ.

If the pancreas is strong and healthy, obesity will take hold and can even worsen; but this will not necessarily lead to diabetes.

If, however, the pancreas is vulnerable and fragile, it ends up becoming exhausted and gives up trying to control blood sugar. When this occurs, obesity is associated with diabetes.

But why does this difference exist between one pancreas and another? Why are some strong while others are fragile and vulnerable?

If you were already asking yourself this question, I've succeeded in one of my goals. And I'm thrilled to be able to give you an answer. The answer will show that, through your dietary choices, you and you alone have the power to determine whether your child will have a strong pancreas or a fragile one.

Only a certain number of obstetricians and diabetologists who focus on gestational diabetes are fully aware of the impact of the maternal diet on the development of a foetal pancreas and the subsequent vulnerability of this pancreas.

Obviously, then, pregnant women are not aware of the facts. How could we expect otherwise? Like all of us, pregnant women are bombarded by flashy, persuasive ads that tell them that there's nutritional value in biscuits that are actually more than 70 per cent ultra-fast carbohydrates.

It took decades for us to succeed in limiting advertising for alcohol and tobacco. Obstetricians have been able to convince their pregnant patients of the importance of avoiding these products. The battle we face now is to do the same for white sugar – **and especially for white flour, which is actually *more aggressive for the pancreas than white sugar.***

To get there, we will look more closely at the glycaemic index. The glycaemic index is a tool that allows us to rate the invasive power of foods containing carbohydrates.

It's comparable to gauging how fast a car can go from 0 to 60.

The fastest carbohydrate is the ultra-concentrated glucose in your blood. Its glycaemic index is 100.

White sugar, or sucrose, is 70 – a high number.

All-purpose flour – what you find in bread or biscuits – is 80.

Now let's return to what happens to those caught in the sugar-insulin-weight gain cycle. With a diet that puts too many sugars in the body, other related phenomena start to appear.

First, persistently high levels of sugar in the blood and in all the organs that it feeds creates oxidative stress: an unmanageable amount of free radicals circulating in the blood.

These waste products are the result of glycation: the binding of a sugar molecule and a protein. They're responsible for aging of delicate tissue, the heart, the kidneys and the skin of the face.

Being overweight also results in adipose cells growing in size, which alters their functioning. This leads to the production of cytokines, which are vectors of harmful inflammation for the organism.

Finally, insulin exhausts the kidney, which causes less effective elimination of salt and uric acid. Too much salt in the blood causes water retention and hypertension; and too much uric acid can lead to stones and gout.

A CRUCIAL POINT

What it means for a food to be refined and industrially processed

We've been talking a lot about foods that are 'refined' or 'processed'. Since industrially produced foods are here to stay, and are even likely to spread, it's important to understand exactly what the terms mean and what they refer to. This knowledge will be especially useful if you're pregnant and eating for two.

Which foods are the ones that are altered and made toxic by the industrial process? From the vast selection of foods available, how do you choose those that are the least processed?

As in our imaginary situation with the packet of biscuits, the following situation will lead to another eureka moment: once you understand it, it will change your entire outlook and permanently alter your approach to food.

The corn process: from the cob to corn flakes

Imagine you're walking through a cornfield and you pick off an ear of corn. Later on, you grill it and eat it right off the cob. In this fresh and natural form, a grilled cob of corn has a low glycaemic index. That's because its strong, dense vegetal texture demands that the body goes through a long, exerting process to digest and break down its fibrous matter. The sugars extracted from the chewed and digested grains arrive in the blood gradually, raising blood sugar very moderately. Insulin secretion, therefore, remains weak.

This digestive journey that starts at the mouth and ends up in the bloodstream can be evaluated on the glycaemic index. This index goes from 0 to 100: 0 is the level of water, and 100 is the level of pure glucose.

On the scale that goes to 100, **the glycaemic index of grilled corn is 36**. Based on the overall parameters, that's a relatively low rating.

Now imagine that, instead of consuming this freshly picked, nicely grilled ear of corn, a manufacturer decides to package it and sell it, in the form of a can of kernels. The manufacturer shells the corn and immerses it in a liquid solution. As the can sits on the shelf, waiting to be sold, the kernels soften as they soak.

This softening of the grain's flesh and skin constitutes the equivalent of predigestion. Your body no longer has to do the work, which makes it that much quicker to digest and absorb the corn's sugars. The sugars therefore arrive faster and in greater number, causing a sharper rise in blood sugar and more secretion of insulin as a response.

When it is shelled and soaked in a solution in a can, the same corn we picked from the field becomes dangerous and causes weight gain. In this form, **the grain's glycaemic index rises from 36 to 50**.

Now let's take the scenario a little further. Another manufacturer takes the grains of corn and decides to make flour from them. The grains are dehydrated and very finely ground; they end up in a beige powder form, which can be used for baking or in sauces. This additional processing further erodes the corn's vegetal structure and reduces the effort necessary for digestion.

In the mouth, the stomach and the small intestine – where the food enters the blood in the form of glucose – digestion and absorption time is reduced yet again. It leads to an even larger irruption of glucose. Blood sugar jumps even more drastically, forcing the pancreas to increase its production of insulin even further.

When rendered as flour in this form, **the glycaemic index of corn climbs even higher than before: it reaches close to 70, which is the glycaemic index of white sugar.**

The final scenario: a third manufacturer takes this flour and makes it into a paste, which is then milled until it's a small fraction of an inch thick. The ultra-fine paste is then cooked until it becomes rigid. Finally, it is broken up into the thin pieces we all know under a common name: corn flakes.

When this final transformation is finished, every trace of the original plant has vanished. The sacrifice is total; a nutritional void remains.

When we consume corn flakes, our digestive tract has almost no work to do. The trajectory from mouth to blood becomes a virtual toboggan ride, with no friction along the way. With the arrival of these sugars in the blood, the pancreas secretes almost the largest dose of insulin possible.

What we see when we look at corn flakes, however,

is merely another food product: fun, crunchy, and with a charming orange colour that's pleasant for kids and reassuring for parents.

And yet the glycaemic index of the corn, now processed to the hilt and transmuted into corn flakes, **has reached a new peak**: between 85 and 92, depending on the country in which it's manufactured.

Remember: we started with a glycaemic index of 36 for corn in its most natural form, when it was still in the farmer's hands. We saw this index rise with each step of manufacturing: 50 when it was canned, 70 when it was made into flour, and as high as 90 when it was turned into corn flakes.

I chose the example of corn because it's a shocking one, and because you, and all consumers, should be aware of the effects of the industrial processing of foods. The same process is involved in almost 70 per cent of the food we eat. The consequences are serious enough that we should be aware of them, at the very least.

I'm certain that this chain of processing is an integral part of the spectacular explosion in weight problems, obesity and diabetes around the world. The birth and advancement of this twofold epidemic are directly correlated to the development of the industrialisation of highly processed foods.

But the impact of food processing alone does not fully explain the epidemic.

A healthy adult's pancreas may be able to tolerate such

an aggressive diet; the same isn't true of the pancreas of a developing foetus. Facing an environment saturated in sugar, this small pancreas will experience faster and more intense growth than usual. The child will be born bigger, and its pancreas will be bigger as well, having been forced to work too hard and too soon. This child will be vulnerable to weight problems and diabetes; and the vulnerability will persist throughout its life.

Let's say the child is female, and let's follow her further. We may get to the point where this girl has grown up – likely to be overweight – and she gets pregnant. During her pregnancy, she will transmit that same pancreatic vulnerability to her foetus. If that foetus faces a nutritional environment as overwhelmed by carbohydrates and processed foods as its mother's when she was in the womb so long ago, the child will be born with vulnerability that has only been compounded by the repetition of the cycle.

The idea here is that, with the invasion of processed carbohydrates, their harmful effects on the development of the foetal pancreas are *transmitted and amplified with each new generation.* This domino effect of the weakening of the pancreas makes its victims more prone to weight gain and diabetes. The proliferation of processed carbohydrate foods has thrown us into a vicious transgenerational cycle that is the cause of the meteoric rise in weight problems.

But here's another shocking thing: it's very easy to stop this escalation. During the two crucial months when the pancreas of your foetus is appearing and developing,

just consume as many natural foods as possible and as few overly processed carbohydrates as possible. That's it. Follow me as we head down the path of learning how.

The appearance and development of the pancreas in the embryo and foetus

This project is concerned with your pregnancy and the pancreas of the child in your womb. Therefore, it's worth knowing how this organ appears during the pregnancy and develops within your baby's abdomen, which is inside your own abdomen.

The appearance and development of the embryo's pancreas, followed by that of the foetus, is orchestrated and regulated by the human genetic code.

It all starts with the meeting of an ovum from the mother and sperm from the father. These two gametes have prepared for their union: they have each shed half their chromosomes so that their merging creates a complete new cell.

This union is the moment of fertilisation; the result is an egg.

Immediately after fertilisation, the egg starts dividing rapidly, at a rate of about one division every ten hours. First, it divides into two, then four, then eight. By the end of the third day, the zygote comprises sixteen small cells: they form the **morula**.

At this stage, these cells are called stem cells, since they are undifferentiated and are still capable of any necessary cell lineage. From this point on, bridges start to form between the cells so that their development is coherent.

At day four or five, we get to the **blastula** stage, which marks the beginning of cell differentiation.

On day six, the developing egg makes a nest in the lining of the uterus.

On day seven, it forms an inner cell mass. This has two layers consisting of different cell types:

- an external part, which forms the skin, nails, tooth enamel and nervous tissue; and
- an internal part, which forms the digestive and respiratory organs.

By the 18th day, the embryo measures: 1 mm.

By the 22nd day: 2 mm.

By the 26th day: 4 mm.

At the end of the first month: 6 mm, which is about the size of a small pea.

During the second month, the embryo starts to take shape externally and positions its internal organs. By the 60th day, the embryo measures almost 3 cm, the equivalent of a grape or a small nut.

Now let's focus on the development of the pancreas.

By the 19th day, two small buds appear on the wall of the intestine: first the **dorsal bud** and, three days later, the **ventral bud**.

By the fifth week, these two buds start to migrate **so they** can meet and merge in the sixth week. Ninety-nine per cent of the developing cells in this pancreas-to-be will eventually play a role in the organ's endocrine function and will produce digestive enzymes; the remaining 1 per cent will be involved in the endocrine function only, with half of them specialising in insulin secretion.

During the fourth and fifth month, the cells that have so far been undifferentiated will come together into little islets called Langerhans. Over these sixty days, these Langerhans disseminate and acquire the capacity to secrete insulin. And that's the way it's been for 200,000 years.

The 'sugars' the mother consumes are digested and then broken down so they can end up in the blood in the form of glucose.

Glucose is a small molecule, so it easily passes through the placenta, transferring from the mother's blood to that of the foetus. But maternal insulin is too big to pass through the same way. That means the foetus must produce its own insulin.

If the mother consumes products that are high in sugars, her blood sugar level will rise. The foetal pancreas will therefore be required to transform this glucose into fat. This leads to weight gain that is proportional to the sugar consumption, and to increased infant birth weight.[11]

By the end of the fifth month, the die is cast. The cells within the Langerhans islets that are responsible for insulin

---

[11] Reece, A. Leguizamón, G. Wiznitzer, A. 'Gestational diabetes: the need for a common ground', *Lancet*, 2009; 73: 1789–97.

secretion have become functional. Their development, and their eventual strength or weakness, depends on the levels of glucose in the maternal blood that reaches the foetus and its pancreas.

Finally, from the sixth to the ninth month, the volume of the insulin-secreting cells will increase, as well as their insulin production.

To summarise: during the two months of the cellular proliferation phase, the beta cells of the pancreas have more power to multiply than ever, and it's during these two months that maternal nutrition must be regulated most carefully.

Conclusion

This chapter was devoted to the pancreas, which is at the centre of the weight and diabetes crisis. This organ should no longer be considered just another part of your anatomy. Getting that idea across is one smaller goal that's part of the greater mission of this book. It's a mission based on hope. By reading on, and carefully, you will become a part of that mission and that hope. As you move through these chapters, you'll see that our shared success would equal a bright future.

The mission is essentially to *protect your child* from a vulnerability that has already entangled 2 billion individuals in weight problems and trapped half a billion in diabetes.

But a related mission is to help you protect *yourself*, by making you aware of the threefold problem with our dietary model today:

- Food has become merchandise, subject to certain market rules: increasing productivity, lowering cost and maximising the incentive to consume.
- Food products have become addictive: their carbohydrates have been concentrated, and their naturally occurring fibres have been removed. As they languish in their industrially concocted nectar, they lose their status as a natural food. The result is that they end up being treated by the reward centres of your brain in the same way as a hard drug.
- Foods that are so rich in these concentrated sugars surpass the functions of the pancreas: an organ designed at a time when these foods didn't exist.

Above all, though, there is one particular moment when the conflict between our ancient pancreas and the sugars of today is most acute, and has the most drastic consequences.

This is the moment when the pancreas starts to form in the foetus's abdomen, itself within the mother's abdomen.

If maternal nutrition is balanced and moderate, in terms of invasive sugars, during this crucial period the foetal pancreas will develop as it should according to the genetic conditions of our species. That means the pancreas stands a good chance of being robust enough to deal with these foods.

If, however, the foetal pancreas appears in an environment filled with carbohydrates and is permeated with maternal blood that often has high levels of glucose, this pancreas will have got off to a bad start; it will be impaired. This pancreas will have a continuing tendency for insulin hypersecretion, a higher birth weight than average, a predisposition to insulin resistance and a propensity for obesity and diabetes.

So join me on a journey to our roots. Our aim is to understand the history of our species, to learn what our genes actually want us to eat, and to appreciate the risks we take if we ignore their demands.

CHAPTER 6

The Genetics of Human Nutrition

What do our genes tell us about our diet and the functioning of our pancreas?

The full response is highly technical. To make it as clear as possible, let's start by looking at what a species is, exactly, and how a species' identity is rooted in its genes.

Each species is determined by a genetic code that differentiates it from other species. Our own genetic code distinguishes us from other living beings by giving us the faculty of being able to create culture and adapt to most situations we encounter. This code is the basic foundation of our humanity.

The importance of the genetic code is not limited to the high-level fields of scientific study. The code is a decisive element in how we manage our lives, in how we can avoid disease, in what we strive for and what satisfies us.

It seems almost ludicrous today, but for a very long time humanity believed that all species on earth were created at the same time. But what we currently know about the history of all the species that have ever lived on Earth falls under a single name: evolution. The then heretical theory was developed (under difficult circumstances) by Charles Darwin and published in 1859. The theory asserted that each species succeeded a previous one, and that species have been evolving, from the time the first viruses came into being until the appearance of humankind.

Specifically, each species follows from an older one, which it has replaced or broken off from. The new species is fully autonomous and the separation is complete when its members can no longer reproduce with members of the former species.

No one knows the meaning of evolution, the ultimate goal. But we do know that evolution advances by increasing complexity. Why does one species come after another? In order to more successfully adapt to the environment, to survive and continue the basic project, which surpasses scientific understanding and pushes life towards an unknown destination.

And for those who want further details: evolution progresses through errors in the transmission of an individual's DNA to its offspring. Poorly transmitted copies generate what are commonly known as genetic mutations, which are normally silent and distributed throughout the entire population.

If some external event occurs that the species is not adapted to, members with the right mutations may have better chances of surviving. These individuals therefore also end up being more likely to reproduce, thereby passing on the mutations to their descendants. Eventually, a family line will break off from the rest of the original species, creating a new species.

This new species' genetic code, which is written into the DNA of each of its members, starts with the following information:

Here's what sets you apart from members of another species. Here's what you will look like. Your eyes will be such and such shape and colour. You will have lungs or gills, skin, scales or feathers, etc.

It also says:

Here's how your body works, how your heart beats, how you breathe, how you control your body temperature, and how thousands of other functions work, with or without your knowledge.

And that's how we come into the world – in an egg, a kangaroo's pouch or another mammal's womb. And an embryo's development takes place according to a very precise and carefully orchestrated process.

One element turns out to be fundamental in the planning for this development. All the animals in the world – including hominids, which includes us – live according to the directives contained in the code of their species.

For social animals, the genetic code tells the species

that living in groups is ideal. The instructions are species-specific: gibbons and wild geese are monogamous; baboons live in harems; wolves live in packs; panthers are solitary. Even the number of individuals in a group or society is anticipated in the genetic code.

Humankind is no different in being bound by this powerful system, which makes us what we are and not one of the countless pre-human and human species that have preceded us.

And this brings us to two issues that concern us here: human pregnancy (yours, in particular) and the formation of the human pancreas (such as that of your unborn child).

For the process of pregnancy, everything is intricately mapped out. It's akin to a musical score that has been read and interpreted for hundreds of millions of years.

The formation of the pancreas is like a single bar on that musical score.

That means that the pregnancy process for a Cro-Magnon woman 40,000 years ago was identical in every way to that of a woman today. Each week brings changes to the embryo and then to the foetus, all leading to birth. Thus, the role and functions of the pancreas too were laid out at our origin some 200,000 years ago and remain the same today. **And that means that, as the pancreas of your unborn child develops, it will follow – exactly – the same blueprint as the pancreas of an infant caveman ages ago.**

I'm sharing this to help you see that the pancreas, which is almost the only agent we have for controlling sugar and fat storage, is not at all adapted to how we eat today. The pancreas is not an organ exclusive to humans, it is found in all wild mammals. These animals, of course, do not consume refined sugars – just as humans, before civilisation began, did not. The idea here is easy to summarise: the blueprint for how the animal or human pancreas functions does not take into account the sugars we consume today – and especially not in the quantity we consume them.

The tension between our ancient pancreas and the modern diet is at its height, and is most dangerous, when this organ first appears. By carefully selecting the right foods to consume during your pregnancy, you hold the power to control that tension. But, if you fail to do so, you may make the violent collision between ancient and modern that much more damaging.

We know that genetics governs our physiology, and that our physiology is adapted to a certain type of diet. And this leads us to see the urgency of protecting the pancreas at the moment when it is formed in the mother's womb.

Let's pause now and look at another example of the relation between genetics and the cultural environment. Breast milk from mammals varies according to species: donkey, cow, human and monkey milk are all different. When the baby bottle started to compete with the mother's breast, the shift prompted a great deal of discussion. Paediatricians began offering their opinions on the issue. Scientists in the United States and in Europe had differing views on the composition of milk – especially regarding the protein content, which was given more importance by Americans than by Europeans.

But it did not go unnoticed, in France, for example, that American GIs abroad were a good 10 cm taller than the French. After decades of debating, it became clear that the best milk for human infants was... mother's milk. In response to this consensus, manufacturers created infant formula. The matter was settled.

This example shows that if a few grams of protein more or less in an infant's milk can make such an impressive difference – creating a taller generation of Americans, for instance – then there is clearly such a thing as an ideal human diet. And it's crucial for you to remember this point during the last six months of your pregnancy – especially during the fourth and fifth months, which are the most critical.

The Great Rift and Hominisation

I considered skipping this section when I was writing the book. However, I just couldn't resist the temptation to share with you what's sometimes considered the greatest story ever told. Besides, it helps me build my case.

It starts with a big question: How did we become human beings?

The action begins in Africa almost 8 million years ago. In the middle of the continent, near the equator, sits the equatorial forest, with its dense and lush vegetation. Among the species of primates who coexist there is a great ape, whose descendants would eventually split into two species: chimpanzees and humans. For the time being, however, the great ape remains safe from predators and unaware of its illustrious future progeny. It has a vegetarian diet, mainly consisting of fruits.

This quiet world is riven in two when a cataclysmic earthquake descends upon Africa like a sword. It creates what is now known as the Great Rift: the continent is severed into two land masses. The eastern part stays in place; the western part collapses.

The forest too is split, separating into a lower part and an upper part. Winds bring clouds and moisture that provide water to the lower part; but the steep elevation of the upper part cuts it off from rain. To the west and to the south, the forest remains hydrated, with dense vegetation. To the east and to the north, however, drought sets in. Vegetation withers, and the region becomes savanna.

Monkeys living in the forested part remain unchanged. But those that live in the savanna, deprived of their trees and fruits, find themselves on the ground, in the midst of tall grasses that hide the horizon from sight.

The only survivors among the newcomers to the hostile savanna are those that carry latent mutations allowing them to adapt to the new conditions. This includes those that can eat animal flesh, live in a pack to defend themselves from predators, hunt, and are equipped with a pelvis that allows them to stand upright to see above the tall grasses.

This upright position, which was necessary for survival

in that environment, was also the key to the later emergence of homo sapiens. The head ended up balanced on the first vertebrae of the neck; it no longer needed to be held in a horizontal position by powerful muscles that surrounded the base of the skull. The skull therefore was able to shift towards the rear, which opened up the space for development of the brain.

Liberated hands were able to be used as instruments for exploring, and fine motor skills could develop. Hands and brain started working together until they were eventually capable of launching a gripped stone so that it could strike prey or predator.

The monkeys that remained in the lower forest evolved very gradually into chimpanzees. Almost 7 million years ago on the savanna, however, the first prehominid species was born, starting with the legendary Pithecanthrope.

The baton was then passed from species to species. Evolution passed by way of the Neanderthals and through two or three other species, until we arrived on the scene.

During this development, the evolving brain went from having several hundred million neurons and a volume of around 100 cm^3, to our 14 billion neurons and a volume of almost 1,400 cm^3.

But it's not so much the number of neurons as the unprecedented complexity of the wiring that connects them that gave birth to reflective human consciousness, giving us not just thought but a unique self-awareness.

Scarcely 200,000 years later, we have become the living

embodiment of the modern human: Homo sapiens. Prehistorians and anthropologists have gathered a wealth of scientific data on our species' lifestyle over time and our progressive occupation of the planet.

From the moment when our species became mature, and in every subsequent generation, the members of our species have had the same, unchanging genetic equipment that adapts us to a certain way of life: that of a hunter-gatherer.

Undeniably, human beings have continued to evolve, particularly in adaptations involving skin colour, hair and other physiological details like lactose tolerance. But the organism has remained essentially the same.

After 190,000 years of hunting, gathering and colonising the planet, humans started to shift into a sedentary lifestyle. We had discovered animal breeding and farming. And for the last 10,000 years, human beings have existed in a civilised state.

I've shared this story not just for your interest, but to help you understand something we tend to forget. It's something that is crucial in order for us to live according to our body's own blueprints. It's the fact that **by nature humans are hunter-gatherers**.

Becoming an adult human in today's world is a very involved process and takes up most of the first twenty years of our life. Unfortunately, it generally ends up with our acting against the grain of our nature. The aspects of our existence that are based on our physiology and the functioning of our body are stubbornly resistant to change: the body is anchored in our genetic requirements.

To illustrate the duality going on, take the example of breathing. Throughout the day, and even more so at night, you breathe automatically, without even thinking about it. But you also have the power to halt that automatic action and stop breathing. Though it's quite obvious, this is an interesting case because it illustrates the confrontation between nature and culture very clearly. Since it's a matter of our survival, nature responds very quickly when you halt your breathing. You experience suffering: sooner or later you give in and nature wins out. You could say the same thing about sleep: it's possible to moderate it, but it will eventually impose its will.

The same goes for any human lifestyle in the midst of a hostile environment, one too far removed from the natural model. I'm thinking here of the consumerist framework of our lives. It's a framework that is deeply damaging to those who are unable to flourish under it. My own experience in treating overweight persons has allowed me to understand and observe the unhappiness that is generated by estrangement from natural satisfactions. This estrangement and the resulting suffering can be tolerated – like holding your breath – but, as always, nature takes its course sooner or later, and demands compensation.

In my area of study, this compensation manifests itself in the compulsion to eat.

For that reason, I'm opposed to the view of certain

psychologists who advocate a balanced diet. After all, you wouldn't suggest to someone who's drowning that they should breathe in a calm, balanced way.

Our world is so hectic, so demanding, that we aren't always aware of the immense changes it has undergone during the last half-century. One of the changes I'm most familiar with is diet. The agri-food industry and food distribution has revolutionised our food supplies. It offers a wider variety of products, but also products that are more seductive, gratifying and addictive. But our digestive system, our absorption process and our metabolism have remained the same as they were when humans came into being. It's this confrontation between our stable nature and a radically evolving culture that over the last fifty years has resulted in an outbreak of 'lifestyle diseases': first and foremost, diabesity, the grouping of excess weight, obesity and diabetes.

These diseases are related to the abundance of food, but it's not so much the overall quantity of food that is to blame. Rather, it's the fault of non-human food products that are so rich in 'sugars' or processed carbohydrates that they surpass the limits of our physiology and have serious impacts on our health.

Insofar as no health organisation has ever succeeded in reducing the consumption of these foods – demand is continually increasing and the selection ever expanding – all these 'sugars' form a united attack on the single thing that counters them: the pancreas and the insulin it secretes.

To deal with this powerful obligation and to continue protecting the body, the pancreas must be healthy, robust and well developed. This robustness depends on the conditions at birth and the first developments of this organ.

When the pancreas is created and as it develops during intrauterine life, it is imperative that it is not disrupted by the excessive presence of invasive carbohydrates. Unfortunately, pregnant women today eat the same foods as the rest of the population eats. This massive influx of sugars does not lead to the robustness the pancreas needs in today's world: instead, it creates an inherent vulnerability to these sugars, a vulnerability that will only worsen over a lifetime.

Still, while the weight and diabetes epidemic is steadily gaining ground, a significant portion of the population is succeeding in escaping it. Their pancreas has avoided that vulnerability.

The goal of this book, aside from giving you enough information to convince you that my approach is sound, is to offer you a specific diet plan for the last six months of your pregnancy, to help you protect the pancreas of your child and prevent the onset of this vulnerability.

If you're a pregnant woman today, there's a good chance you're between twenty-five and thirty-five, and your mother is between fifty and fifty-five. That means when your mother was born, around 1965, the prevalence of childhood obesity was at 3 per cent; it's at 18 per cent today, and it's likely to reach 25 per cent by 2020. Childhood obesity rates have doubled every ten years for the last thirty years.

If you can, ask your grandmother whether she ate differently during pregnancy to how you do. You'll see that the difference has less to do with the quantity of protein- and fat-heavy foods and more to do with the current omnipresence of industrially manufactured invasive carbohydrates.

Once we become clearly aware that our new dietary model is responsibility for these health epidemics we face, **we must protect the foetus at the decisive moment where the pancreas is formed and starts to develop.**

To get to that point, however, we still have to dig a little deeper into the evolution of the human diet, to see how pregnant women ate in the 190,000 years before civilisation, and then compare that to the last fifty years.

Cordain's study: 229 hunter-gatherer societies examined

In 2000, an American team undertook the largest synthesis to date of the diets of hunter-gatherers who lived in natural conditions in the twentieth century. This synthesis completed and confirmed the data gathered by prehistorians on archaeological remains.

This study examined the diet of distinct isolated populations living on different continents, in order to find what foods were constants. The underlying premise was that what *varies* in terms of diet from one group to another is a matter of *culture*, and that what is *universal and unchanging* is *natural*. Here's what the research found.

On average, across all the populations studied, two-thirds of the calories consumed were of animal origin, and one-third were of plant origin. Now let's look more closely at this average to examine the nutritional categories contained in their diets.

Of these populations, 20 per cent consumed **only** products from hunting and fishing; their diet included only proteins and fats and almost no plant matter and therefore no carbohydrates. No population studied was strictly vegetarian.

To be more specific, here's the comparison between the diet of a hunter-gatherer and the diet of a modern Western human:

Proportion of three nutrients

	Proteins	Fats	Carbohydrates
Current Western diet	15%	33%	52%
Hunter-gatherer diet	27%	43%	30%

This suggests that, no matter where they lived, the first humans – natural-living humans – generally consumed:

- twice as many proteins as today's humans;
- 30 per cent more fats than today's humans; and

- almost half as many carbohydrates as today's humans, and no fast carbohydrates – and certainly no processed and refined carbohydrates, the kind that have been industrially mass-produced for forty years.

It's important to realise that not only did primitive humans consume few carbohydrates, but also the carbohydrates they consumed were among the slowest that have ever existed: they would occasionally find carbohydrates in acidic berries and wild grasses packed with fibre. These few carbohydrates are even slower than those we call 'slow sugars' today.

I've already mentioned the concept of happiness held by the Inuit, who live in cold regions where no vegetation grows during the seemingly endless winters. Paul Emile Victor, who lived with Inuit people for a winter, spoke of how they find plants when summer returns: 'They gathered wild vegetable sprouts like wild celery and especially cranberries, the only fruit produced on Greenlandic soil, and they made preserves using seal oil for winter provisions.'[12] This shows us it's possible to live seven months a year spending most of the time hunting under hostile conditions and maintain our body temperature and brain activity in extreme temperatures without ingesting carbohydrates other than those found in seal liver.

---

[12] Guillaume, Jean, *Ils ont domestique plantes et animaux. Prelude a la civilisation,* (translation) Quae Editions, 2011

Today we live in warm homes and have a highly sedentary life, but somehow – against sound judgement and scientific reasoning – we continue to actively promote a diet containing 55 per cent carbohydrates.

The Cordain study concludes that, regardless of the foods available in their climate and their culture, humans in a natural environment instinctively follow a similar proportion of the three universal nutrients.

If we accept the fact that our genes govern our physiology and our metabolism, if we accept that they orient our choices, our dietary and metabolic needs, then the primitive human's diet, generally consisting of fresh food, should serve as our primary source of inspiration.

The universality of Cordain's study shows that the basic structure of the human diet was modified with the emergence of civilisation. When humans took up livestock and agriculture, the door was opened for carbohydrates, for grains such as wheat, rice and corn. But back then, these grains were nearly wild and were consumed in their natural state.

This original explosion of carbohydrates brought the first change to the perfect balance of the three nutrients, proteins, fats and carbohydrates. But while this added amount of carbohydrates imposed a heavier workload on the pancreas, it did not exceed the organ's limits.

After the introduction of grain farming, carbohydrate consumption remained stable, quantitatively and qualitatively, for thousands of years. The really radical disruption of the human diet came when industry, economics and advertising joined forces to create, manufacture and promote industrially processed, refined and concentrated carbohydrates.

The widespread distribution of these foods had two major impacts on health.

1) They put too much demand on the pancreas and exceeded its ability to function properly. Overwhelmed by the influx of glucose, the insulin secreted by the pancreas has no choice but to neutralise the nutrient by transforming it into fat.

2) The massive influx of highly concentrated carbohydrates like table sugar or modified white flour – foods invented by humans and not anticipated in our genetic makeup – are able to set off the brain's reward circuits, producing massive seduction and consumer addiction.

To understand the effect produced by the refining and concentration of carbohydrates, consider what happens to a grape when fermentation transforms it into wine. The case of beets is even clearer: a perfectly harmless vegetable that, through industrial concentration, is transformed into white sugar.

We have to distinguish between foods that nourish and satisfy us and those that intoxicate us and distract us. A manufacturer's goal is to produce as much as possible, at the lowest cost, and to generate the highest profit margin possible. To achieve this, manufacturers aim to produce food products that are malleable, alterable and made addictive so that consumers keep coming back for more.

Let's take stock of what we've considered so far. We have examined the role and the functions of the pancreas and its role as regulator of your blood sugar level. We've learned that, without the pancreas and its insulin, a dose of glucose higher than 10 grams per litre of blood would be fatal. Today, however, it's nothing unusual to consume 100 grams of these invasive sugars. To deal with this perpetual and potentially deadly threat, the pancreas plays a role it has never played before in the animal kingdom: **it transforms sugars into fats.**

In this chapter, we peered through our species' 200,000-year history. We saw that, for the first 190,000 years, the consumption of carbohydrates was very low and had no impact on the pancreas.

For 9,950 of these years of the last 10,000 years, those spent living in a civilised mode, humans have increased their consumption of unprocessed carbohydrates. This created a strenuous amount of work for the pancreas, but one that the organ could still tolerate.

In the last fifty years, there has been a definite rupture in the human dietary model, with the emergence and ever-accelerating expansion of industrially transformed carbohydrates. This explosion took place between 1965 and 1970: the public became intensely concerned about fats, which opened the door for sugars to fill the void.

That was the moment when the adult human pancreas became an overworked and threatened organism. But this threat becomes supercharged when it targets the emerging and developing pancreas of a foetus.

In the next chapter, I will present a monumental scientific discovery, one that has revolutionised biology. Exciting research is uncovering new facts that we would never have imagined in the past. **What we're finding is that the environment can intervene on the expression of our genes.** This intervention can take place any time, but especially during an individual's growth period – and, most of all, in that magic moment when our genetic score is articulated, during our life in the womb.

CHAPTER 7

Epigenetics

We've come to the point when all the information we've explored in the previous chapters can be assembled and used as a tool for moving forwards. The things we've learned will make the task at hand clear and simple.

And, if you start by accepting the gravity of the problem, you'll also be ready to adopt the strategy I've created as a response.

We began by focusing on the seriousness of the weight and diabetes crisis that faces us today. Within the span of just two generations, these previously rare conditions have simply exploded. They're now an epidemic that affects all of civilisation, and the leading cause of mortality around the world.

Health organisations have offered unhelpful tautologies

and simplistic explanations to explain the crisis. To summarise: people are eating too much and not getting enough exercise.

But using the 'calorie balance sheet' doesn't explain much; it tells us only *how* we gain weight. It's essentially the same as explaining alcoholism by saying that people drink too much.

My goal has been to lead us to the **why** – the deeper, hidden explanation for excess weight and diabetes. It's the only explanation that really gets us anywhere, and the only one that we can truly use to defend ourselves.

The explanation – the **why** – has two parts. One is social, and the other is nutritional.

• The social aspect: our consumption-based modern lifestyle seems to be more rich, stimulating and innovative than any that has come before. But that lifestyle has been shaped by the *economy* – and it's fundamentally intended to *serve* the economy. To keep creating profit, consumers must keep consuming.

  A remarkable form of culture has emerged to encourage this consumption. This culture distances us from our deep human needs, and puts artificial needs in their place.

  The lifestyle we have today is disconnected from our original, natural model. Our lives have become artificial and cold. We've ended up pervaded by unhappiness; to feel better, we self-medicate with food and entertainment.

- The nutritional aspect: the key here is the recent invasion of industrially created foods. These foods are constantly becoming more intensively processed – they're hyper-refined and high in 'sugars'. The food selection on our shelves and in the advertising we see demands more from our pancreas than it can handle. That's because the pancreas was 'programmed' *back when these foods didn't even exist.*

Chapter 5 was devoted to the pancreas and the insulin it secretes. This organ is at the core of my argument, and of the project that I believe in so deeply. It's essential that we understand the role of the pancreas, and the part it plays in weight gain and diabetes. It will help you to protect yourself and, more importantly, the child you will bring into the world.

If you choose to follow the plan in this book, your child will be born with better protection against excess weight and diabetes. And an even better result is possible if a large number of pregnant women follow the plan. The results would quickly give clear and objective proof that the project is completely valid. Then more people will be helped, and the benefits will snowball.

Chapter 6 focused on a story that's as exciting as any you'll find in a novel: the story of the beginning of our species. Our long, amazing journey started in the equatorial forest of Africa, from the last ape to the first hominid. Species followed species, until you and I emerged: homo sapiens.

The pre-humans and the humans that followed them primarily subsisted on proteins and fats. For 7 million years, the only carbohydrates our ancestors ate came from vegetables, leaves, roots and, during very short seasons, berries and wild grasses.

So, if our organs are oriented towards specific functions (which is true of living things generally), then our need for carbohydrates is actually very minimal. The existence of essential amino acids and fatty acids proves that proteins and fats are vital nutrients – we need them to live. Conversely, the lack of the equivalent acids for carbohydrates tells us that there *are no such things as essential carbohydrates*.

This is particularly significant for the pancreas. The organ was designed when the world was sugarless, and it now faces an invasion of the worst forms of sugar – intense and violent forms, which neurologists consider the same as drugs.

Here's a basic fact that's essential to human life. Without the pancreas (and insulin-dependent diabetics effectively live under this condition), blood glucose is:

- harmful above 1.40 grams per litre; and
- fatal above 10 grams per litre.

To protect the body from the recently appearing dietary threat, the human pancreas is forced into a mission for which it wasn't designed. It must fight a lifelong battle against a deadly poison. To do so, it sends out a foot soldier to transform the poison into fat.

However, the lobbies for the white sugar and white flour industries are finally losing ground. It's happening very slowly, as it did for tobacco. The sugar-based industries are still doing everything they can to stem the popularity of diets low in invasive carbohydrates.

Here are the basic elements of the epidemic of excess weight and diabetes (insofar as it affects *adults*):

- a diet that's been invaded by industrially processed sugars;
- an overwhelmed pancreas that was designed millennia ago;
- a species whose diet contained almost no carbohydrates until the advent of civilisation; a species that has been consuming 'sugars' for just fifty years; and
- a strong craving for sugars **that give us pleasure in a world that makes us feel bad** – that provide a way to compensate for our lack of fulfilment (but make us fat in the process).

All of these elements help us understand the epidemic. And yet, they don't give us a *complete* explanation for the incredible *scope* of the epidemic.

Seven questions remain unanswered. Trying to answer these questions led me to the solution contained in this book's plan.

1) The first question led to a turning point in my thinking and became the inspiration for the project of this book. What caused the rise in average infant birth weight between 1970 and 2006?

2) How can we make sense of the incredible speed at which the epidemic has spread, affecting billions of people and resisting our every attempt to curb it? The basic explanation health authorities give for the massive and rapid invasion of weight problems is that we're eating more and moving less. This explanation just isn't sufficient.

3) What explains the increase in gestational diabetes, a condition that affects women in the last months of their pregnancy?

4) Similarly, how is it that we all share the same culture, which presumably determines our diet, while only a portion of the population is affected by obesity and diabetes?

5) Why is there now an undeniable connection between obesity and diabetes, while they were once distinct conditions?

6) Why does insulin work differently in various individuals who don't have diabetes? Why do some people secrete more insulin than others for the same quantity of sugars consumed?

7) Why do some people have cells that become resistant to insulin more quickly? They may never become resistant, some do slowly, and some do quite quickly (and the latter group is becoming more numerous).

As these questions loomed, a number of determined and curious researchers and practitioners started focusing on the concept of **vulnerability**. But what was the *origin* of this vulnerability? The answers remained elusive.

Then finally, a breakthrough: an explanation was found that would seriously disrupt one of the main dogmas of biology of the last two centuries. A new branch of biology was developed: *epigenetics.*

It all started thirty years ago, when Dr David Barker, a British epidemiologist, found extensive evidence that the risk of death from infraction was correlated with birth weight, and much more so than all other known risk factors in adulthood.[13]

It was the first time that a link had been found between an event in early life, birth weight and a health risk that affects adults.

The new theory, however, was not immediately welcomed. Some claimed that the research was poorly done. The idea was ridiculed; those who developed it even had their sanity questioned. But other scientists were interested. They took the research further, and found more support for the ideas. As they did, the theory started to have a greater impact.

What had Barker said that was so shocking? His fundamental observation – based purely on facts – was that, during pregnancy, the foetus can be affected in a way that will change its birth weight and leave it with a lifelong vulnerability to certain diseases in adulthood.

---

[13] *Lancet*, 5 October 2013, vol. 382, No. 9899, p 1170

A new branch of science was born, a powerful and incisive discipline that we now know as epigenetics. Since then, researchers have been pouring into this field – a field that offers hope for explaining the origin of some of the most widespread diseases affecting civilisation.

A growing number of studies and research – some focusing on animals, most being epidemiological studies on humans – have confirmed it: the maternal diet and a woman's psychological and emotional environment during pregnancy can increase the risk of her child developing a susceptibility to one of the many chronic illnesses that are a byproduct of modern civilisation.

Genetics and epigenetics

Before epigenetics was discovered, genetics reigned supreme – there was no competition.

Genetics is based on Darwin's theory of evolution, Mendel's three laws of inheritance, and the discovery of chromosomes and the double helix of DNA.

Darwin's theory centres on the occurrence of small transcription errors in the genome that are passed on from one generation to the next. The errors result in random mutations. These mutations are passed on only if they prove beneficial for the next generation.

Of course, this evolution usually takes place over hundreds of millions of years. The process can't adapt to the sudden and frequent changes we face in our chaotically shifting world today.

But, incredibly, it's been discovered that some genetic evolutionary changes have occurred over *just one generation* – changes that would normally take more than a hundred generations to develop.

This contradicted the dogmatic belief that acquired traits can't be transmitted. To our great surprise, we have found that events and environmental pressures can in fact modify how genes function.

Understanding epigenetics

Epigenetics is best understood as a way that the genome takes a kind of 'pilot fish' approach.

The genome is like a mothership (to change our metaphor): it's large and powerful. When it needs to make adaptations quickly, it sends out a faster, more agile escort ahead of it.

The genome is made up of DNA, which is shaped like a double helix. A single DNA sequence contains a virtual library of information. Genetics is the study of genes; epigenetics focuses on the modulation of the *action* of these genes, but not modification of the *sequence*.

Genes are almost unalterable; they change only through profound and stable mutations. Epigenetic modifications, on the other hand, are reversible.

Let's consider a simple example of epigenetics at work. All bees in a hive start their life as larvae. But some will end up becoming workers, others will become guards, others will be foragers, and just one will be queen. *And it all depends on how they are fed.*

Here's another example, an even clearer demonstration of what distinguishes epigenetics from genetics. A turtle egg will become a male or female adult turtle *based solely on water temperature*: that's epigenetics at work.

These examples show us that, while genes carry a message, the environment can cause *modifications* to that message, to adapt it to the needs of the species. Here's another metaphor: while genes are the motor, the epigenome is the rudder (or the shock absorbers).

We could also think about epigenetics in terms of a symphony by Mozart. The majestic piece of music is mapped out by the composer's hand; eventually, it becomes a part of our species' heritage. But, in the years that follow, any performer or conductor can bring their own sensibility to the piece, adapting it to the aesthetics of their own time and place. The audience brings their own context to the experience too, interpreting the music in their own way.

In the broadest terms, then, that's what epigenetics is and how it occurs. Thousands of researchers have been researching this fascinating branch of science, and they've shared their findings with the world.

So why do you need to know about it?

The answer will become clear soon enough. Suffice to say it's no smaller matter than changing the entire life of the child you're bringing into the world. And when I say *the entire life*, it's no exaggeration.

From the moment your oocyte detaches from your ovary and encounters a man's spermatozoa, an egg is formed. It

146

will divide and re-divide *fifty-six times* in the process of becoming a child.

As these fifty-six divisions unfold, epigenetics can intervene to amplify or weaken the unfolding of the genetic message, if the environment demands it. And the role of epigenetics doesn't stop when a child is born; it develops throughout their life, following the same principles. Epigenetics may be a recent discovery, but its effects are very real.

Here's a simplified explanation of how epigenetic effects occur.

Your DNA contains your design; the plan for how you'll operate is inscribed on a double helix coded with just four letters: A, G, C and T. These are the nitrogenous bases: adenine, guanine, cytosine and thymine.

To intervene on this fundamental text and make modifications, epigenetics uses two methods: methylation and histone modification.

DNA methylation

In very simple terms, a molecule is methylated when a small appendage is added that modifies its shape. This appendage, which plays a role in epigenetics, is known in chemistry as methyl radical.

For example, let's take cytosine, one of the four base types of the genetic alphabet, and follow it through transcription.

Like all molecules, cytosine's activity is determined by its shape, the same way the shape of a key determines which door it can open. To alter the activity of cytosine, epigenetics modifies the molecule's shape by adding a methyl radical in a specific place that will change the molecule's message.

This task is carried out by an enzyme, methyl transferase, which dislodges the cytosine hydrogen molecule on its fifth summit and replaces it with a CH_3 methyl radical.

You might be surprised that such a small change can affect the relay of information. But it can, and the same goes for all types of communication. Think about what would happen if you called your mother on the phone and asked for 'Tom' instead of 'Mom'. All it takes is one single syllable to completely derail the original message.

Transcription regulation by histones or 'Transcription regulation by histone methylation'

The centre of operations is the cell.

Inside the cell is the nucleus.

Inside the nucleus are chromosomes.

Each chromosome contains a DNA double helix, coiled around a spool of histones to form a nucleosome. Groups of nucleosomes form chromatin – the raw material of chromosomes. The spool of histones is what gives DNA its density and structure. By changing this density – by increasing or reducing the amount of histones – the genetic message can be modified.

Anatomically, the histone has a tail that extends outside of the nucleosome.

Epigenetic changes are made to the histone tail in

order to affect the relay of information. There are four different types of histone modifications, but acetylation and methylation occur most frequently. Acetylation is used to promote gene expression, while methylation is used to repress it. Just as a piano's notes can resonate loudly or softly depending on how it is played, genes can be either intensified or muffled.

By combining methylation and histone modification, we arrive at epigenetic modulation of the genetic code within the nuclei of the cells.

The parent's genomic imprint

We're also starting to discover that epigenetics operates at a level that transcends a single individual's development. Further upstream, it also intervenes on the genes of each parent separately, before they even meet. This intervention takes place on the genes carried by the father's sperm and the mother's oocyte. All these markings combined make up the parents' genetic imprint.

This means that the father, who plays no physiological role in pregnancy, through information transmitted via his sperm, can effect changes on a child developing in the womb.

Conclusion before we look at how the plan works

First, I want to emphasise an important point. When excess weight, obesity or diabetes is already a problem and its onset can't be avoided, what I've argued all my life is still true: anyone who wants to lose weight can do so. But, aside from surgery, the only way is through diet.

Losing weight is neither simple nor easy, and its process can often be inconsistent. But for those who really want to do it and continue the project into the future, it's very possible. Unfortunately, this crucial motivation is systematically sapped, even demolished, by the enormous resources of the agri-food industry: particularly sugar and flour producers.

As a physician, my training has always focused on eliminating suffering and disease. A simple sore throat is something I can't ignore; any other doctor would say the same. My response is that much stronger when a life is in danger. And if hundreds of millions of lives are threatened – what then?

For this reason, and for the honour of playing a part in an important mission, I've designed and created this plan to help stop the obesity and diabetes epidemic, by approaching it from a new starting point.

This plan aims to slay the monster of excess weight and diabetes by attacking it and neutralising it at the moment when it's most vulnerable: just when it's beginning to form. This decisive moment is the time when the foetus's pancreas begins to emerge and develop in the mother's womb.

This approach is based on scientific data from epigenetics, which I certainly did not invent. Hundreds of thousands of studies have already established and confirmed the theory behind epigenetics. My goal is to apply that theory to solving the weight crisis here and now.

The experience I've gained in the field and the views of the best experts in this new scientific field have convinced me that the plan must succeed. There are three reasons for this.

It is simple, healthy and centres on your main job during your pregnancy: maintaining a good, healthy diet.

The plan is also intended to reach the ears of a woman who is unlikely to be misled: a mother-to-be whose instincts are in a heightened state.

And finally, the agri-food industry that thrives on excess weight and hinders the treatment of the problem will no longer take the risk of openly opposing the project: doing so could mean alienating its own consumers.

My message for mothers-to-be

If you're just beginning a pregnancy, you're at the start of the most amazing project a human can carry out: creating new life.

Over the nine months to come, an essential organ will start to form in the body of your unborn child: the pancreas, which will regulate its glucose throughout its life.

Up until the end of the third month, this pancreas, nothing more than an outline positioned on the embryo, is made up of cells that are not yet able to produce insulin. It's during the next two months, the fourth and fifth, that the cells acquire this ability. It all takes place according to an extremely precise and carefully orchestrated design that has been unchanged since our species emerged.

This design accounts for everything, but for one critical omission: it is not prepared for foods that have never before existed in the history of human life. These new foods are the processed 'sugars' in our daily diet.

Epigenetics was discovered thanks to the wisdom and curiosity of researchers who were determined to understand crisis situations that occur when the environment creates a problem that genetics can't handle.

Thirty-five years after David Barker's original observation, it is now undisputed that the environment can modify the expression of genes throughout an individual's life.

We also know that the more environmental disturbance occurs at an early stage of life, the more its effects are felt later on.

The most critical period of all is the period of pregnancy. Today we have an impressive body of research proving that the genetic score, which orchestrates the development of the pancreas, is modified by the 'carbohydrate storm' that rages through the mother's diet.

During the fourth and fifth month, the foetal pancreas starts to secrete insulin. While that ability is forming, it meets this powerful adversary, which it will spend the rest of its life trying to neutralise: excess glucose that reaches the foetus via the mother's blood. Imagine an everyday situation: an expectant mother prepares a plate of white rice and a glass of fruit juice, or picks up a little sandwich on white bread from the supermarket.

In the mother's blood, glucose levels can easily rise to 1.40 grams per litre. This blood travels to the foetus, which has started developing insulin-secreting cells. However, the small foetal pancreas doesn't have enough insulin to neutralise the sudden influx of sugar. Because the foetus is still developing, it reacts by producing more insulin-secreting cells so it can release a sufficient amount of the hormone. The resulting increase in insulin transforms the sugar into fat and causes the foetus to grow. This causes a higher birth weight. This disturbing phenomenon has been happening regularly for two generations now.

And here's the crux of the problem. Over time, your child's pancreas will continue to hyper-secrete. This makes them predisposed to excess weight, insulin resistance, diabetes and metabolic syndrome. And, as we have seen, these pathologies have grown exponentially in the past decade.

Can this catastrophic phenomenon be stopped?

The only answer is that it *must* be stopped. But how?

Again, a single answer: it can only be stopped by tackling the root of the problem. This root is the overwhelming flood of invasive and processed sugars in the foetus's food environment.

You are the only one who can take action and help prevent these pathologies by choosing your diet wisely during the next sixty days. The solution is simple, logical and healthy for both you and your child.

The three-phase protection plan in this book follows your pregnancy calendar and varies according to the level of risk for each period.

1) The first trimester: the pancreas is not secreting any insulin, and your diet has some flexibility.
2 The fourth and fifth month: the pancreas begins to secrete insulin. Risk is at its highest in this phase. If you watch your diet with extreme care, the benefits will be huge.
3) The final four months of pregnancy: the risk decreases somewhat, and your diet regains a bit of flexibility.

Today it is recommended that pregnant women refrain from smoking or drinking alcohol. These recommendations make perfect sense, and women generally follow them.

For this project, you are asked to make a much smaller sacrifice, with a different focus.

By protecting your baby's developing pancreas, you will also be protecting their future. What's more, your own health will benefit, as this diet will reduce your risk of gestational diabetes, a phenomenon often associated with an excessive consumption of invasive carbohydrates.

And it's not just about your own family. You'll be fighting for a cause that concerns the future of all human beings. It's no exaggeration. A large number of women adopting my prevention method could easily lead to a shift for our entire species.

As we have seen, for the past thirty years the general population – pregnant women included – has been eating too many processed sugars. As a result, children are being born with a pancreas that has had to work too hard too soon, and carry a vulnerability to excess weight.

What's more, when these children grow up and pass on the trait to their children, this vulnerability is exacerbated. This trans-generational relay might explain the astonishing increase in obesity.

I'm not the only one taking on this daunting challenge. Countless researchers have rallied around epigenetics, compelled by its strong scientific foundation.

The next chapter therefore examines the scientific evidence for epigenetics.

CHAPTER 8

Scientific Evidence

A s I've mentioned, this project – like all innovations that threaten the interests of the powerful – will be met with opposition and controversy.

Some will argue that such a large-scale, world-changing project cannot be developed by a single person. And they're right. In this short chapter, we'll look at the scientific basis of my proposition.

As you'll see, I'm far from being the only one investigating this threat. I'm fascinated by epigenetics, but countless other researchers have also converged on the field. With its strong scientific foundation, it has truly revolutionised biology.

Since the turn of the century, epigenetics has been the focus of more than 130,000 research articles on developmental programming. This vast body of work reflects our increased interest in epigenetics, with its various sub-disciplines, as well as the possible effects epigenetics will have on our future.

Furthermore, the 2013 DOHaD World Congress (17–24 November) brought together more than a thousand researchers in Singapore.

For those interested in learning more about epigenetics, please consult the references and further reading at the back of this book. It contains only a small fraction of the massive amount of literature on the field, with a focus on the most concrete and least technical articles.

The first epigenetic studies

In 2001, paediatricians from the Robert-Debré Hospital and the French National Institute of Health and Medical Research (INSERM) in Paris formed the Haguenau cohort, a study that explored the data of 27,000 individuals born in Haguenau, France, between 1971 and 1985. Among this group, 734 individuals had been born full term with a low birth weight. They became the focus of the study.

The subjects were twenty-two years old on average and in good health. Importantly, none suffered from type 2 diabetes. However, they were twice as likely to have disturbances of blood glucose as the control group. Some even presented early signs of insulin resistance, a characteristic of type 2 diabetes. The only variable was their low birth rate.

Eight years later, in 2009, these same subjects were

invited to undergo a second medical examination. Those who had a low birth weight were still relatively healthy, but their insulin resistance had increased compared to the control group. Excess weight and obesity were also common among the individuals with low birth weight.

In the wake of Barker's first observation, different researchers started to scrutinise other existing data. Statistics about the offspring of women who had survived long and intense famine because of World War II revealed something extremely interesting.

During the Dutch famine of 1944–45, adult rations fell to 580 calories per day – just a quarter of a healthy adult's average food intake. Unsurprisingly, malnourished women gave birth to underweight babies. When girls born during the famine eventually grew up and had children of their own, their infants were also underweight, despite having been born under normal dietary conditions. This cycle was perpetuated over many generations. The fundamental discovery here was that changes caused by a **hostile environment** could *alter the genetic programme* – not only in individuals but across generations.

Over-nutrition and malnutrition

The field of epigenetics emerged from Barker's observations on malnourished mothers and the below-average birth weight of their children. Later, studies were done on birth weights during wartime food shortages – the data was abundant and easily accessible.

As the epidemic of excess weight, obesity and diabetes continued to spread in the 1970s, more important studies were conducted on the phenomenon of above-average birth weight. Again and again, it was found that nutritional deficiencies had directly affected newborns' birth weight.

Professor Yajnik, a leading expert in diabetes research, found that at one time the number of malnourished people in India far exceeded the well-nourished, and vastly outnumbered the overweight. Today, however, the situation has reversed itself: the country faces a high susceptibility to obesity and diabetes. Yajnik made a table that breaks down the proportion of what he calls 'the thin and fat'. His conclusion? Pancreatic vulnerability is acquired *in utero*, both through malnutrition and over-nutrition.

Today, the Western world no longer suffers from hunger, and industrially processed food has flooded our diet and insinuated itself into our nutritional model. And, for the past ten years, most developing countries have gone in the same direction. In these countries, there's a strong correlation between poverty and excess weight. The explanation for this relationship is simple: carbohydrates are the least expensive of the three nutrients to manufacture, and the only one that causes insulin secretion.

Epigenetics and current events

In 2010, **King's College London collaborated with the Beijing Genomics Institute (BGI)**, a leading global genomics organisation located in Shenzhen, China, to set up a $30 million project called Epitwin. The massive study will examine how the lifestyles and eating habits of 5,000 twins lead to differences in gene expression. They hope to learn how twins' identical genomes can change over time due to epigenetic effects. Greater knowledge of these epigenetic effects may make it possible to develop medication to inhibit genes associated with heart diseases, obesity, diabetes, osteoporosis and even longevity. Until now, such studies have focused on handfuls of twins; the Epitwin study will multiply the number by 1,000.

'Today, abundance is prevalent, not famine,' says **Professor Claudine Junien from the Necker-Enfants Malades Hospital in Paris**. 'We've seen that a quarter of women of reproductive age are overweight or obese. *Increases in food consumption and decreases in energy expenditure alone cannot explain the current epidemic of obesity.*' [14]

In 2011, science writer Joël de Rosnay called recent discoveries in how species adapt to their environment through epigenetic changes 'the great revolution of biology of the past five years'. [15]

It's a concept that proves that, when it comes to genes, 'fatalism' is at least partly false.

Dr Jennie Brand-Miller, a specialist in infant nutrition

---

[14] *La Recherche*, April 2012, 463, p 48

[15] Rosnay, Joel de, 'La grande revolution de la biologie de ces cinq dernieres annees – pas dix, vint, trente: cinq dernieres annees'.

and a world authority on the effects of carbohydrates on children's health comments that:

'Maternal nutrition is more important than we ever imagined. Life inside the womb is a critical period for metabolic programming that influences a baby's cell types, cell numbers, body composition, hormonal feedback, metabolic activity and appetite. Our food supply and dietary recommendations should be based first and foremost on the needs of pregnant women. If we cover them, we automatically cover everyone else. They should not be seen as the exception to the rule (and given nutritional supplements). We now also know that different patterns of growth have long-term effects on the risk of specific diseases. If growth is restricted, there is a higher risk of abdominal obesity, cardiovascular disease and type 2 diabetes as an adult. Over-nutrition – seen for example in maternal diabetes and obesity – is also linked to increased risk of obesity in adult life. The positive news is that we know that interventions in pregnancy are probably more effective than later interventions. So we have to give Mum and her unborn baby much greater focus.' [16]

Research and studies on epigenetics and type 2 diabetes

This line of research emerged because the traditional model of genetics is unable to explain the causes, the enormous

---

[16] Miller, Jennie Brand, Marsh, Kate and Moses, Robert, *The Bump to Baby Low GI Eating Plan*, Hachette Australia, 2012

increase and the astounding spread of type 2 diabetes in children. Researchers have been focusing on determining how pressures from the dietary environment can influence the appearance of this condition during pregnancy.

For the team of **Professor François Fuks at the Université Libre de Bruxelles**, 'there is no room for doubt: the epigenetic modifications in the cells of the pancreas that produce insulin are associated with the disease'. [17]

Dr Marie Aline Charles, research director at INSERM, a French health organisation, commented on Professor Fuks' studies: 'This type of study shows us clearly that, during foetal development, something happens that affects us for years and can alter our future.' [18]

Dr Charles' own work currently focuses on the effect that the father's obesity can have on children's health. While research tends to be more concerned with the mother's diet, a number of studies have shown that the father's diet also plays a role in 'programming' diabetes in the foetus.

Mark Hanson, Professor of Foetal and Neonatal Physiology, London University: from October 1993 to December 1999, Professor Hanson examined umbilical cords from 300 infants born in the 1990s, and uncovered a wealth of data on the mothers' diet during pregnancy.

Nine years later, he measured the fat mass of these children: 'those whose mothers had a very unbalanced diet

---

[17] *La Recherche*, April 2012, *op cit*

[18] Charles, M.A., L'unite mixte Ined-Inserm-EFS

in pregnancy are bigger, and one of their epigenetic marks was well altered at birth,' [19] he says.

In 2011, a major international study, led by Professor Keith Godfrey from the University of Southampton, showed that, during pregnancy, the mother's diet can modify the unfolding of the genetic programme that steers the infant's development. 'We have shown for the first time that susceptibility to obesity cannot simply be attributed to the combination of our genes and our lifestyle, but can be triggered by influences on a baby's development in the womb, including what the mother ate. A mother's nutrition while pregnant can cause important epigenetic changes that contribute to her offspring's risk of obesity during childhood.' [20]

The study showed that epigenetic changes observed at birth significantly predicted obesity in early childhood, from six to nine years old.

The authors show that, to prevent childhood obesity, we need to focus on the mother's diet during pregnancy. Their evidence confirms that all women of childbearing age should have access to a diet that's adapted to our current information, so that the next generation can be protected from the risk of conditions such as diabetes and heart disease that frequently follow obesity. *

Along with the **WHO, DOHaD (International Society**

---

[19] 'Medicine and Research', Seminar 12 of the IPSEN Foundation, Endocrinology Series

[20] Source: University of Southampton, 'New link between mother's pregnancy diet and offspring's chances of obesity' study, 2011

for Developmental Origins of Health and Disease) is the leader in research on the foetal origin of chronic diseases of civilisation. Their goal is to fight against the relentless march forward of such diseases: hypertension, obesity, diabetes, cancer, Alzheimer's and allergies. These conditions are the cause of more than half of all recorded deaths each year: 35 million now, and likely to reach 42 million in eight years.[21] Clearly, the economic costs will end up exceeding every health budget imaginable.

DOHaD argues that the current approaches to fighting the scourge are doomed.

Mark Hanson, president of DOHaD, put it this way:

'Until now we have only addressed the patients with disappointing efficacy. People are made responsible for what they consume and their lack of exercise, they are accused of "gluttony" and "laziness". The genetics they share is overestimated; the genotype accounts for less than one-third of the variability at birth, mostly due to gene-environment interactions, provided by epigenetics.'[22]

DOHaD believes that it's now possible to change the direction of these alarming statistics, so long as we intervene early, before the risk has even appeared. This action should be targeted at young adults that are at reproductive age

---

[21] Hanson, M., Gluckman, P., 'Developmental origins of non-communicable disease: Population and public health implications', *American Journal of Clinical Nutrition*, 2011, 94, p 1754-8

[22] 'Medicine and Research', Seminar 12 of the IPSEN Foundation, Endocrinology Series

and mothers during pregnancy and throughout infancy. The essential thing is to share the invaluable findings and get the greater public involved. The gap between scientific knowledge and consumer awareness is still far too great.

The WHO's 1,000 Days[23]

The culmination of this international action is the WHO's programme, 1,000 Days. Here's the organisation's objective, in their words: 'These 1,000 days, between the very beginning of the pregnancy and the end of the second year of the child, constitute a window of sensitivity of our organism. A period where the environment imprints on our genes sustainable epigenetic marks that will condition the future risk of disease of an individual.'

The goal, in other words, is to fight against the relentless spread of chronic diseases that the WHO believes present a serious threat.

I'm deeply impressed by the ambition and enthusiasm behind the project, which aims to prevent all chronic diseases of civilisation. But I fear that the Herculean task will take too long to carry out.

To the great credit of the researchers and health organisations involved, the revolutionary plan has a solid foundation. But, as it gradually comes to fruition, time will continue marching on. Meanwhile, in France alone, 800,000 children are born each year whose diet (apart from

---

[23] See www.thousanddays.org/

an absence of alcohol and tobacco) is no different to that of the rest of the population.

The crisis is worsening at a much greater rate in highly populated developing countries such as China, India and Africa, where diabetes and obesity are affecting children and adolescents at an ever-younger age.

As for my role, I'm limiting my focus to the sphere I know best, the one that's closest to my heart. It's a project that's already immense – almost at the edge of impossibility. It's simply to promote a diet that protects the foetal pancreas.

My mission and my approach therefore remain centred on the same fight I've long been waging against excess weight, obesity and diabetes, which together constitute the leading risk of morbidity and mortality.

Each year, millions of children are born with epigenetic markings that predispose them to excess weight, diabetes, suffering and disease. For this reason, I believe it's crucial to act quickly. The evidence is clear; there's so much to gain *and nothing to lose.*

As a doctor and nutritionist, I've spent my life as a therapist in direct and daily contact with patients whose lives have been afflicted by their excess weight, and even more by their diabetes – and more still if they are obese.

From what I see, the situation must change here and now.

The risk or danger from taking up the battle? None.
The benefits to be gained? Immeasurable.

The French author Paul Valéry coined a phrase that I

carry with me every day. I think of it as a powerful call to arms for those ready to join me in fighting this epidemic:

The wind is rising; we must attempt to live!

How the plan works

A word of warning

The recommendations of this plan do not constitute a diet – above all, it should not be considered as a diet for losing weight.

This warning is worth thinking about. I know, from experience, that any project that fights obesity and diabetes is a threat to powerful interests; it will meet criticism, hostility and fierce resistance.

I'm aware of this fact because I myself experienced this hostility when my books and method started being used by millions of people.

All members of human society are part of one species, originating from the same genome. And, just as each conscious individual has a subconscious that orients them towards survival, society also has a kind of subconscious of its own.

As members of a society, most of us care about the weight crisis and its effects on health – on a *conscious* level. We also care about the 2 billion people affected, and about the enormity of resources health agencies must spend to fight the problem.

Subconsciously, however, other motivations are at play. The overwhelming priority of society today is economic growth. No matter how high the cost of the pandemic, it will never equal the profits of the two top economic players: the agri-food industry and the pharmaceutical industry. Both profit from the existence of weight problems. The agri-food industry makes its profit by manufacturing enticing and addictive products that cause weight gain. The pharmaceutical industry makes its fortune by treating the avalanche of health complications caused by those processed foods: weight and diabetes.

Although my weight-loss method received a great deal of attention several years ago, I want to be very clear that the plan in this new book is in no way aimed at making you lose weight. Its sole purpose is to make pregnant women understand that some foods that appear perfectly tolerable throughout much of their lives are actually very dangerous during a short time for a gestating foetus. The vast majority of women today know that drinking fizzy drinks and eating corn flakes and sweets is less healthy than eating, say, a salmon fillet with asparagus. But a great many women still indulge in the less healthy option – after all, it won't kill you.

The problem, however, is that during pregnancy a mother-to-be is eating for two. She is likely to be unaware that some of the foods that she loves – foods that are pushed relentlessly on TV – are harmful for her unborn baby. And yet it's obvious that an adult's body is stronger and more resistant than that of a small child. Just look at the labelling on any box of medication: dosage varies with age.

So, this plan is not intended to help you cut calories, and even less to help you lose weight: its aim is to help you reduce your consumption of certain foods that may disturb the immediate development of the foetus.

I also know that pregnancy and the development of future offspring are sacred topics for many. This sensitivity may drive people to be more circumspect with any new approach. I would expect no less – especially since the project laid out in this book and the plan that follows from it has an entirely different scale to that of a weight-loss plan that targets individuals.

If, as I fervently hope, a high number of women end up adopting the plan, they will drastically reduce the amount of highly processed foods they consume. And those who make their living from these products – directly or indirectly – will find that change very hard to accept.

But there's also a comforting thought. I firmly believe that pregnant women, imbued with hormones and that mysterious force we call 'the maternal instinct', are able to withstand the persuasive powers of marketers. They have an innate ability to discern what is good for their unborn child.

The big industries may be able to fool a great many consumers who are unable to see through the fog of misinformation – but it's more difficult to fool a mother-to-be who carries a child in her womb.

This project has a chance to help make a significant change at a moment when more and more voices are telling us that sugar should not be part of a human diet. The time is right for my message to be heard. And I'm addressing this message to all mothers: the origin of our human world.

The main objective of the plan

The plan is founded on a major scientific breakthrough: epigenetics. This field has taught us that powerful new environmental pressures are capable of modifying the genetic code. And this modifying action is more effective, more intense, when it surrounds a crucial, precarious moment during intrauterine life.

Epigenetics gave me the keys to understanding the incredible recent increase in infant birth weights. During adult life, this increase develops into a vulnerability to excess weight and diabetes.

The vulnerability is a hidden weakness in a person's body that will cause it to deteriorate faster than those without it.

It's common these days to learn that car manufacturers are recalling cars that came out of the factory with some vulnerability in their components or their systems. Often it's an error in the information system that manages a chain of mechanisms. It's a good analogy for what happens when a pancreas develops vulnerability during its formation in the womb.

The vulnerability is centred on the pancreas of the child you're carrying, and affects its future production of insulin. The way you eat during your pregnancy will have a decisive impact on the construction of that tiny pancreas. If you limit or eliminate the consumption of industrially processed carbohydrates, your child's pancreas will be fundamentally strong and healthy. But if you abuse these foods, you'll raise your blood glucose levels too quickly and powerfully, you'll disrupt this organ's development. And this organ is the only thing that protects us from diabetes and weight gain.

Nine months: it's a long time, and yet remarkably short. To give the developing pancreas the most effective protection possible, specific measures are required that target the most sensitive periods for the maternal diet. Providing a clear road map that targets the most critical periods will help mothers-to-be remain focused and motivated.

The message is simple and clear: avoid consuming too many processed carbohydrates; these foods excessively raise the level of glucose in the maternal blood, which reaches the foetus through the placenta.

After a balanced meal – appetiser, main course, dessert – your blood sugar can reach 1.40 grams per litre. If the meal is rich in invasive carbohydrates, your blood sugar can climb even higher. It will climb higher still if you indulge in snacks that are high in 'sugars' – for instance, a muffin on your way to the office.

Another important point: it's commonly believed today that there are two families of carbohydrates: invasive ('fast') carbohydrates and gradual ('slow') carbohydrates. The difference is thought to be based on their chemical structure and their glycaemic index.

This oft-used index measures the ease with which foods containing carbohydrates are digested and assimilated, from their being chewed to the arrival in the bloodstream (it's a little more technical and complicated, but that's it in a nutshell).

Health organisations are finally calling for moderation in the consumption of carbohydrates with a high glycaemic index, such as white sugar, white flour and all their derivatives. They also consider 'slow' carbohydrates to be 'good' foods, and recommend consuming starches at every meal – even for diabetics.

The glycaemic load of foods

Warning: If distinguishing among carbohydrates based on invasive power is valid, it's qualitative and not quantitative. In other words: it doesn't account for the *portion* consumed. In fact, it all comes down to the dose.

The glycaemic index is helpful only if we compare equal quantities of carbohydrates. Let's consider the example of legumes, which are one of the foods that are lowest on the glycaemic index.

When you consume 100 grams of lentils, digestion and absorption is slow and uneven, which raises your blood sugar only moderately. The effect on the pancreas and its secretion of insulin is therefore weak.

If you consume 300 grams of lentils, carbohydrates still arrive in your blood slowly, but in a more concentrated way. Appearing all at once, they have a stronger impact on your blood glucose. The *quantity* alters the situation.

Because of this, we need to take another, more complex index into account: the glycaemic load.

Here's how the **glycaemic load** is calculated for a particular food:

glycaemic load = [glycaemic index x quantity of carbohydrates per portion of food (g)] / 100

Let's break that down:

1) Start by calculating the quantity of carbohydrates in the portion you're investigating. Be careful: don't mistake the amount of carbohydrates for the weight of the food that contains them. For example, 100 grams of biscuits may contain 45 grams of carbohydrates, or 65, or 70. Check the nutritional labelling carefully.
2) Multiply this quantity by the glycaemic index (between 0 and 100).
3) Divide the product by 100.

What can we learn from the result? Let's see together.

Example: 100 grams of French bread

The glycaemic index is 80
In 100 grams of French bread, there are 50 grams of carbohydrates
Its glycaemic load would be 80 x 50 = 4,000
Divide by 100 = 40

Example: 300 grams of tomatoes

Glycaemic index 35 x [4.6 g/100 g], so for 300 g = 483 divided by 100 = 4.8

How to classify glycaemic loads:

- 10 or under: low glycaemic load
- 11 to 19: considered moderate
- Over 20: high glycaemic load

Examples of glycaemic loads:

- 200 grams of cooked couscous: 31.2
- 200 grams of spaghetti: 35
- 20 gummy bears: 29

As you can see, 200 grams of couscous or spaghetti has the same effect as 20 gummy bears.

Conclusion: while you may hear that you're supposed to eat starchy foods with each meal, pay close attention to the quantities you eat. Remember that all carbohydrates, from honey to lettuce, from white bread to green beans, end up in the blood sooner or later in the form of glucose.

To put it another way: don't make the common mistake of thinking 'If the glycaemic index of this food is low, I can eat as much as I want, whenever I want.' Don't rely solely on the glycaemic index, especially during pregnancy; consider the quantity as well.

Periods during intrauterine life when the foetal pancreas is extremely vulnerable

For those of you entering pregnancy, that huge event in a woman's life, and who want the best for your child, this book will help you avoid the risk of your child being born with a **vulnerability** to excess weight and diabetes. This vulnerability may severely impair their life.

The goal of the plan I'm presenting to you here is to prevent a pancreas – an organ programmed to develop in the context of a low-carbohydrate maternal diet – from being subjected to a diet rich in carbohydrates, *particularly* addictive, industrially processed carbohydrates.

The push and pull between the genetic score and the nutritional environment triggers an epigenetic adaptation. This adaptation changes the plan for the pancreas's development. The pancreas is forced to make adjustments; in doing so, it becomes distorted. Given the significant importance of the pancreas in managing sugars and fats, the vulnerability caused by this alteration will greatly affect the future health of the adult-to-be.

What I want to do with this plan is give you the ability to prevent this vulnerability from occurring.

Any time you consume sandwich bread made with flour that's been stripped of every trace of vegetable matter; or corn flakes, for which the same is true; or biscuits that mainly consist of this same flour and white sugar; or a handful of gummy bears; or a fizzy drink, consider the concrete facts. These foods were not meant to be part of the human diet.

If you're *not* pregnant and you eat this way regularly, it will lead, sooner or later, to weight gain. If you keep up that diet over the years, you will continue to gain weight, and you will start to tire your pancreas. Eventually, the organ may fail, triggering diabetes.

You may not notice the effects until ten or twenty years have passed. But if you're choosing this sort of risky diet, know that you will be affected. A price must be paid eventually – but it's you and no one else who will pay it.

If you're pregnant, however, it's an entirely different story. Each second, an embryo and subsequently a foetus creates millions of new cells. These organise themselves to form a human, with a predetermined shape and 'operating system'.

If today's computers were millions of times faster and more powerful, we could read a human genome and deduce the form and functioning of the developing child. The design is incredibly precise; the slightest grain of sand is unable to slip into the gears of our machinery, which has been working for some 200,000 years. Unfortunately, the average diet of a mother today introduces more than a grain of sand – it's more like an entire dune in the Sahara.

In the next section, I've located and ranked three distinct periods during your pregnancy based on the risk that your diet may present to the development of your child's pancreas.

The first three months of your pregnancy

During the first trimester, the pancreas emerges in the embryo's abdomen. But at this point it isn't yet connected to what the mother eats and is incapable of reacting to it.

Here's precisely how the pancreas develops in the first three months.

The pancreas starts to develop from two microscopic buds. A ventral and dorsal outline appears, on the 26th and the 29th day, respectively.

In the fifth week, the ventral bud moves towards the dorsal to connect with it, passing underneath and behind it. The two buds collapse and merge during the seventh week.

This future pancreas is thus well into its development. But it has not yet acquired the feature that interests us most here: the ability to secrete insulin.

Does this mean that epigenetic mechanisms are not active during this period? Not really; genomic imprinting takes effect during this period. This phenomenon, which we have been studying and learning more about for twenty years, shows us that epigenetics plays a role at this stage too.

Normally, the spermatozoa from the father and the oocyte from the mother are wiped of any epigenetic markings that may have occurred over their lifetime.

This removal takes place so that a new individual can be born. However, it has been found that some parental genes are not entirely unmarked, and these markings can have an influence on the genes' expression. As we have seen, the epigenetic markings are made via methylation or histone modification.

While we're well aware that the mother's diet and history

of weight problems leave their mark on the foetus, we have also found that the father's diet and weight history have an influence. It's during the first trimester that that influence may take effect.

However, the effects of this imprinting exceed the scope of my project here. While I'm convinced that the most effective approach is educating parents facing a pregnancy, I also know from decades of observation that it's surprisingly difficult to get the facts across. Practising strict self-restraint in a world of excess, while our appetites are manipulated by those who feed on addiction, is a praiseworthy goal – but it's also a utopic dream.

When it comes to dietary habits, I know from experience that only extremely simple strategies – painless and extremely direct – will work. So, if you're planning your pregnancy well in advance and you're in a position where you can wait until the right time, you can start now: prepare a diet that *focuses on controlling the quality and quantity of industrially processed carbohydrates.* If you're at the start of a pregnancy now, focus on that nine-month period – especially the fourth and fifth month, when things are most critical. This **sixty-day window** carries the biggest risks, but it also offers the greatest opportunity to have a positive effect.

The fourth and fifth month

We've come to the key moment in plan that lies ahead of you: the sixty days when everything we've looked at so far takes on a heightened importance, when it all fits together and becomes actionable.

Why are these months so important?

Because that's when your child's pancreas makes its official appearance and starts to function. During these two critical months, its development follows, with incredible precision, a 200,000-year-old design. This design leads to the creation of a fully formed organ (and the star of this book): a pancreas that possesses an endocrine function. During this period, it will secrete its first drops of functional insulin.

And that's why these eight weeks of your pregnancy should be seen as the time when the future of your child's pancreas hangs in the balance. It's an extremely short time when the human genetic programme enters into open conflict with a diet that is partly *in*human.

You may have noticed by now that I'm repeating the same theme again and again. I'm willing to take the risk of repeating myself; the stakes are simply too high to leave anything to chance. It's essential that readers are informed, and convinced. Learning happens through repetition, and the lesson at the heart of this book is absolutely crucial.

If you're a woman in the twenty-first century and you've become pregnant, the child you're carrying will develop according to a programme that has not changed since the origins of our species. Our design was created at a time when the carbohydrates we consumed mainly consisted of leaves and roots, and a few berries and grasses during the short season when they were available. And, even more significantly, invasive carbohydrates – those that come in boxes or packages and fill up the overstocked aisles of our supermarkets – *did not even exist.*

And despite this fact, at the most crucial moment for its development, the little pancreas your child is forming will face – in unprecedented amounts and at an overwhelming frequency – an enemy that it will fight for the rest of its life. This enemy is a glucose level that the organ does not yet have the means to neutralise.

To illustrate the situation, here's a comparison. Paediatricians recommend against parents starting their child walking too early. Why? Because the bones of the lower limbs need to calcify and become solid enough to support the body's weight. If parents rush the process, the baby will learn to walk earlier than most, but will risk having bowed legs. Like the foetus's pancreas, the bones of the lower limbs are particularly vulnerable for a time.

Of course, you can still live a pretty good life with bowed legs. The same result is not as certain for a vulnerable pancreas – especially in a world where food processing is constantly reaching new heights.

If a developing pancreas forms a vulnerability from an early stage, the child may face a serious condition for life: the tools needed to deal with blood glucose will be inadequate.

If, during the fourth and fifth months, the foetal pancreas is flooded with maternal glucose, epigenetics intervenes. It does so by intensifying the development of the pancreas and increasing the number of cells that secret insulin.

The more invasive sugars you consume, the more glucose will end up in your blood; as glucose levels rise, the developing child's pancreas produces more insulin cells and secretes more insulin accordingly up until childbirth. Insulin can only neutralise the glucose by transforming it into fat; that means the child will be born bigger, often exceeding 3.5 kilograms.

And it doesn't stop there. After birth, the growing child will be at an increased risk of remaining overweight – from six months to five years old, and on through puberty and adolescence. This acquired vulnerability also increases the child's risk of becoming insulin resistant at an early age, of continuing to gain weight and of acquiring diabetes.

However, YOU hold the power to fend off the crisis, by stopping the dangerous carbohydrate storm that wreaks havoc on a developing pancreas.

All you need to do is modify your intake of the most aggressive and invasive carbohydrates for two months.

Two months.

TWO MONTHS.

So much is at stake that I believe you'll be able to reduce your intake of 'processed sugars' easily and painlessly. By processed, I mean industrially produced – refined, altered and stripped of their fibre. Specifically, I mean white sugar, extracted from red beets, and genetically modified white flour: both are nutritional wastelands.

If you follow the plan in this book – **if you simply eat**

the way your grandmother did when she was your age –
you yourself will become healthier, but, more importantly,
you'll be protecting your child from a threat that is far
from disappearing.

The problem is, we're all surrounded by the same
dietary culture; **we've come to think it's normal.** In
truth, it's anything but normal. Our potent and highly
artificial modern food products have existed for barely two
generations – only fifty years. That's why comparing it to
your grandmother's diet makes a great deal of sense.

It's worth noting that this epigenetic adaptation isn't
limited to weight, obesity and diabetes – it's an element in
all the diseases of civilisation. I chose to focus my work on
these particular conditions for two reasons. First, because
nutrition is my area of expertise, an issue I've worked
on intensively and studied deeply. Second, because the
problem affects fully one third of humanity.

And amazingly, this epidemic – as vast as it is – is in
some sense in your hands. What you need to do in response
requires neither frustration nor deprivation. And a proper
start to your child's life is at stake. I believe that you'll find
the challenge thrilling, and the result incredibly rewarding.

With that in mind, please read and reread the preceding
chapters until you fully grasp the facts and the scientific
basis for this project.

Above all, let your instincts guide you.

Processed sugars are your enemy, and insulin is a friend –
such a friend, in fact, that it saves your life each time you eat

a carb-heavy meal. But it does so by making you gain weight. As an adult, you have the chance to cope; but your unborn child doesn't have the same tolerance. Their back is to the wall. You have only one task: avoid consuming excessive amounts of these 'sugars'. I think you'll accept the challenge.

The last four months

Over the last four months of your pregnancy, the developing pancreas becomes mature and functional, and starts secreting insulin.

If the expectant mother hasn't been careful with her diet and (like most of us) has consumed more invasive sugars than our genetic programming prepares us to deal with, the child she carries will enter the sixth month with a pancreas that is *already enlarged* and *secreting insulin before schedule*.

If the diet remains the same during these last four months, the unborn child will continue to secrete insulin and to gain weight as a result.

As this situation occurs, other parameters come into play, such as maternal weight and personal or family propensity for diabetes.

If the expectant mother began the pregnancy overweight or obese, or if she has a history of insulin resistance, she's at risk of developing gestational diabetes and causing her child to be born with a birth weight higher than 3.5 kg.

But if she has carefully controlled her consumption of invasive sugars:

- her child will have a pancreas that is in accordance with our genetic programming;
- she herself will have gained the appropriate amount of weight – normally between 10 and 13 kilos;
- she won't have created the conditions for gestational diabetes; and
- her child will have a birth weight under 3.5 kg and won't be vulnerable to excess weight or insulin resistance, nor to metabolic syndrome or diabetes.

Summary and conclusion

The first trimester ends with the transition from embryo to foetus; it's one of the strangest and most miraculous moments in a human life. But we're only partially concerned with this period here, since the pancreas-to-be is still nothing more than an undifferentiated mass. However, there's one principle that your obstetrician would surely agree with: avoid gaining too much weight at the start of your pregnancy – especially if you're overweight to begin with.

For the fourth and fifth month, your mission is to keep your blood glucose level between 0.8 and 1.10 grams per litre. Blood sugar isn't just acceptable at this level – it's essential. Above that, however, it becomes harmful. By limiting your intake of invasive sugars, you'll effectively cap your blood glucose levels. That means you'll avoid creating a vulnerability that will be a danger throughout your child's life.

You've probably noticed that there are women who are lucky enough to find 'invasive sugars' fairly unappealing to begin with, who have no taste for biscuits or sweets, and aren't drawn to white bread or white rice. These women inevitably have a normal weight, and neither they nor their children have much need to be protected.

For the countless others who do have an attraction to 'fast carbs', a choice must be made. On the one hand, the fleeting pleasures of carbohydrate rewards; on the other, the extraordinary project of bringing a child into the world with the proper equipment.

For twenty years, obstetricians have asked their patients to stop smoking during their pregnancy. Most patients have accepted – including those who had been unable to quit for their own sakes.

More recently, the recommendation of abstinence was extended to alcohol. For some years now, it has not been a question of reducing alcohol intake but of eliminating it completely.

My goal (and I'm not alone) is for dangerous sugars to be put in the same category as alcohol and tobacco, at least for the fourth and fifth months: the most critical months for the development of the foetal pancreas that has such an important role to play.

We often hear nutritionists telling us that it's misguided to demonise any particular food; and they're right. But first we have to agree on what counts as food. Is it merely anything we can put in our mouth?

Consider the case of chocolate. In the seventeenth century, cocoa was a medication that you'd only find at the apothecary.

Another problem is that any definition of a food should include an account of quantity. Beets are a natural food; the white sugar extracted from them is considered food as well. But is sugar still food in the amount of 100 grams, when you need 1250 grams of beetroot to produce that much of it?

The same is true for grapes. The wine extracted from grapes is clearly a food; but, above a certain quantity, consuming wine is not about quenching thirst, nor even enjoying the taste; it's about getting drunk.

When it comes to carbohydrates, the food industry uses two basic ingredients to produce an endless number of derivatives: white sugar, which is industrially extracted from beets, and highly modified white flour.

These two ingredients are used for biscuits, sweets, breakfast cereals and the massive array of snack foods that are overtaking our diet more each day. All these seemingly diverse foods have something in common: they deliver extremely powerful sensations. Moreover, their digestion and fast absorption violently raises the concentration of blood glucose, delivering a psychotropic and comforting effect.

Leading diabetologists ask their patients to carefully avoid 'invasive sugars'. My view is that the same recommendation should be given to the obese and not just the diabetic.

And a message for those who would defend invasive sugars: saying that a food is dangerous is not the same as demonising it.

And now, a message for pregnant women: consuming certain foods during the two months when your child's pancreas emerges and takes shape can have dire consequences. On top of the pleasure of eating healthily, you'll be giving the child a pancreas for life.

For these last four months:

- If you haven't been careful with your diet in the two preceding months, the foetus's pancreas will have more cells than it should. Starting from the sixth month, these cells will multiply less, but they'll increase in size. Together they will form a pancreas that is larger, richer in cells and secretes more insulin – effects that will have their own consequences.
- If the two previous months were navigated carefully, the ones to come will continue on the same path, towards the development of a strong, healthy pancreas. If you've followed the guidance in this book, you'll probably start to notice that the foods that are harmful for your baby no longer hold the same appeal.

During the last months of your pregnancy, you'll enter a period of insulin resistance. This is perfectly natural. The purpose is to allow a pregnant woman to store fat more easily as she brings her pregnancy to term. But because we're no longer living under the hunter-gatherer conditions of our ancestors, this insulin resistance may accelerate your weight gain.

Here again, the remedy is the same: mastering your blood glucose by limiting the foods that raise it too high, too often.

And now let's turn to your road map for pregnancy.

CHAPTER 9

Your Daily Diet

Diet during pregnancy

The first three months

During the first trimester of your pregnancy, your baby doesn't have a functional pancreas and is unable to secrete insulin. There are no special guidelines for you to follow at this stage.

Simply follow the 'Five Basic Steps', in this next chapter, which focuses on the fourth and fifth months.

And of course, follow the advice that your doctor gives you. Quit smoking and abstain from alcohol; walk for half an hour a day.

Even more important, try to avoid stress. A number of researchers have been working on the epigenetic role of stress during pregnancy. Weigh your daily stresses against the wondrous event of your pregnancy. Don't let the insignificant threaten the essential.

That's all I ask of you for the first three months. Apart from that, use that time to prepare for what comes next.

The fourth and fifth month

We've reached the eye of the storm, the most important moment for the project at hand. It's here that your intervention will be most decisive.

During these two months, your baby's pancreas will undergo a rapid metamorphosis; the organ will undergo more transformations than it will during the rest of its lifetime. Its little cells, which had been inactive, undifferentiated and unspecialised, will acquire the capacity to secrete insulin.

As soon as it gains this capacity, the emerging pancreas is capable of capturing glucose in your shared blood, in real time. And it attempts to respond by secreting the necessary amount of insulin.

If, with the information you possess, you wisely decide to reduce your consumption of highly processed carbohydrates, the little pancreas will mature according to the genetic programme that directs all its operations.

If, however, your diet contains too many foods with a high glycaemic index, you will be forcing the cells of the budding foetal pancreas to work at maximum capacity to manage the excess glucose. This abnormal pressure – which isn't planned for in the programme – leads to a weakened pancreas that will no longer be able to operate as it's supposed to.

During these crucial two months, here are the consequences that can arise and that you must stay diligent to avoid:

- A pancreas with too many cells and that secretes too much insulin.
- A foetus that grows faster than expected and is born with excess weight. (This was the symptom that led me on the path to developing this plan.)
- Too much demand on the body's cells, which must start submitting too early to the orders they'll continue receiving from insulin for the rest of their lifetime. Permeated too early, these cells get worn out faster from having to soak up excess glucose. This exhaustion opens the door to insulin resistance, weight gain and obesity, often followed by metabolic syndrome and diabetes.

Together, these parameters make up the vulnerability that is appearing in a growing number of infants today.

I also believe that the global spread of this acquired vulnerability points to a way of understanding the explosive spread of the weight, obesity and diabetes crisis.

Ultimately, however, the only link between our dietary environment and your unborn child's developing pancreas is you and the food you choose to consume.

It's all up to you, to make the right choices during a very

short period, to avoid flooding your unborn child's body with harmful glucose.

You have the power to prevent this vulnerability from taking root.

Now it's time to learn what you need to do.

I've already mentioned the Five Basic Steps to take over the first three months. You'll probably be surprised at how simple they are, and how easy and self-evident. These steps alone are enough to mitigate some of the risk.

Because the steps are as important as they are simple, I suggest you follow them throughout your pregnancy, from the first day to the last – and later than that, if you're breastfeeding. **I suspect you'll find them so easy, and the results so positive, that you'll end up following them for the rest of your life.**

My assurance comes partly from my own life. I've adopted these basic principles for myself; the rest of my family has too. I try to share them with everyone who's close to me, and with anyone who cares about the health and well-being of themselves and their family.

I can't overstate the extent to which I believe invasive carbohydrates or 'sugars' go against nature. Their explosion throughout our food landscape coincides to a very exact degree with the weight, obesity and diabetes crisis.

So you can imagine how much that nutritional artificiality can damage a foetus that's developing according to a design created 200,000 years ago.

The Five Basic Steps

1) Replace white sugar (sucrose) with coconut sugar (extracted from the coconut flower)

French and European health recommendations are clear on the subject of sweeteners but no study has actually been conducted in pregnant women. But I do not want this limitation in pregnancy to suggest that I am opposed to the use of sweeteners. I say this, and I repeat it, since I am a nutritionist, the danger of sugars is assured, serious and alone responsible for the double epidemic of obesity and diabetes that has already affected 2 billion people in the world. Whereas no health authority in any country in the world has ever questioned any risk associated with the use of sweeteners.

A recent study showed that the more sugary fizzy drinks a woman consumes, the higher the risk of premature delivery. The same relationship has not been observed with light soft drinks.

I've already mentioned a certain line of thought that says it's wrong to prohibit any food absolutely, because no food is dangerous in moderation. There may be some truth to this. But for every person who can stop at one square of chocolate or a single cigarette after a meal, there are countless others who end up unable to resist the desire to consume further.

There are also some foods that lend themselves to moderation better than others. It's not very often you hear of bulimics overindulging on leeks, for instance. And remember, white sugar shouldn't properly be considered a food. It's a product that has been intensely condensed, refined and concentrated. The substance it has become borders on the pharmaceutical. We know – and it's finally starting to be said – that the refining and concentration that takes place during the extraction of sugar allows it to activate reward centres in the brain, the same way 'hard drugs' do.

Here's a shocking example. Several years ago, a French researcher was studying rats that were regularly administered cocaine.[24] By the fifteenth day, the rats had developed the habit of going to one corner of their cage for their dose of drugs. Then a second bottle was introduced, in the other corner of the cage. The rats hesitated at first, then tasted a bit of each. In the end, they ended up favouring the new bottle. **The contents of this bottle were nothing but water and white sugar.** Look for the video online; seeing the rats aggressively feed from the bottle and hearing their desperate sounds will really make you think about the effects of sugar on an adult animal. The effect on a foetus between the fourth and fifth month is far more than anyone would want to risk.

To conclude on this important issue, my advice is that as there are no large-scale studies on sweeteners

---

[24] Lenoir, M., Serre, F. and Ahmed, S.H., 'Intense sweetness surpasses cocaine reward', *PLoS One*, August 2007, 1; 2(8). Universite Bordeaux, CNRS, UMR 5227.

and pregnancy, I caution you during pregnancy to avoid sweeteners and to sweeten your diet only with coconut sugar, an authentic fruit sugar but whose glycaemic index is very low and has no action on the glucose rate of the mother and that of the baby.

I repeat to avoid any misunderstanding: do not use sweetener during pregnancy and instead use sugar extracted from the natural coconut flower.

2) Switch from white bread to whole-grain

When we're talking about white bread, we're talking about any bread made with **industrially processed white flour**. Wheat is a wild grain that was domesticated when humans became sedentary. From the dawn of civilisation until the mid-twentieth century, the species of wheat we've used has evolved slowly. Over the last fifty years, however, agriculture has revolutionised the process; we have multiplied the number of crossbreeds and hybrids in order to create more manageable species. Wheat is now the modern cereal that has been most extensively modified by humans.

Industry has pushed the transition even further, by subjecting flour to physical and chemical treatments to make an ever finer powder that can be sifted.

White flour is therefore very poor in fibres, minerals and vitamins; but it's very rich in starch. Processed white bread made from this flour is a true nutritional void, and the carbohydrates it contains are extremely invasive. Let's recall a powerful fact we saw earlier: the glycaemic index for industrially produced white flour and the bread made with it is 80 – *higher than that of white sugar itself, which is 70.*

And what about whole-wheat bread? If the bread is made industrially, it's often *reconstituted*: it is white bread to which wheat bran has been **added**. This artificial recomposition is nothing more than a marketing ploy: it's a blending, not a binding. The combination of flours breaks down during the digestive process. The white flour advances much more rapidly than the wheat; it detaches from the stomach and races towards the small intestine, then enters the bloodstream. This causes a steep rise in blood glucose levels. The bran arrives later, after the violent battle has taken place: the white flour has already been transformed into glucose, and insulin has been summoned to do its job in response.

The situation is very different for whole-grain bread, which contains the entire grain, ground up but with no parts sifted out. The end result is flour made up of particles of flour and bran that are fused naturally and have not been separated. Whole-grain flour therefore contains all the grain's fibres, as well as the germ. The latter turns rancid very quickly, which means the artisanal bakers who work with it have to grind it quickly and use it all up each day.

Whole-grain bread has an extremely low glycaemic index (35 to 40), which means only a moderate amount of work for the pancreas during its ultra-sensitive development phase.

During the fourth and fifth months, treat yourself

to organic whole-grain sourdough, prepared the old-fashioned way: slow-fermented with stone-milled flour, kneaded by hand.

3) Switch from white rice to whole-grain brown rice

Rice is a cereal grain from Asia that started to spread across the world in the twentieth century. It's now used so widely that we have all the facts on the healthy way to consume it.

During your pregnancy, I recommend you switch from white rice to whole-grain brown rice. The reasons are similar to what we saw with wheat. The white rice we see today has been husked and polished to improve its yield and make it more attractive. This process has eliminated much of its antioxidants and all the fibres that slowed down its absorption.

In a recent epidemiological study published in the *British Medical Journal*, a medical team from Harvard reviewed a high number of studies that monitored more than 350,000 people in the United States, China, Australia and Japan over a long period. They found that eating white rice raised the risk of developing diabetes by 25 per cent. The risk was as high as 55 per cent for people in Asian countries who consumed large amounts regularly.

If you eat white rice often and in large quantities, it's essential that you switch to whole-grain brown rice during those crucial two months – and you should stick to a normal-sized bowl. If you're not great at self-restraint, switch to whole-grain basmati (it's not easy to find, and it's a bit more expensive than most other kinds but it is worth it).

4) Switch from white pasta to whole-grain pasta

There are two typical kinds of wheat used for pasta. Hard wheat is used for dry pasta, and soft wheat is used for fresh pasta and Asian noodles.

If it's hard wheat, it's more resistant to being broken down during digestion and enters the blood more slowly than soft wheat. That tells you that you should opt for pasta made from hard wheat.

However, whole-grain pasta is really your best choice, and for similar reasons. It's made with wheat kernels that still have their outer covering. They're richer in vitamins and minerals, but it's their fibre content that really counts for you, because of their ability to stem the invasive power of sugars.

The ideal, then, is pasta that is both whole-grain and made from hard wheat.

But that's not your only concern. Consider how pasta is cooked as well. Follow the Italians' example and cook it *al dente* ('firm to the bite'). Remember, the general rule is that anything that attacks a food's resistance – in this case, cooking – is a form of predigestion. That means less work that will have to be done during digestion, and faster absorption and more drastic blood glucose elevation.

And don't be fooled into thinking that whole-grain pasta is less delicious than white. Many who eat it regularly find it denser and more rustic, with a more satisfying chew.

This recommendation isn't aimed at you as an adult unless you're overweight or predisposed to diabetes. It is aimed at your unborn child, whose pancreas needs to be protected as it navigates the most crucial part of its development.

5) Switch from fruit juice to whole fruit

Why? For the same reason again: to avoid the products that industries turn from natural to artificial. Under the pretext of making a food more 'convenient' – more practical, comfortable and easy to consume – the food industry took natural fruit, squeezed it and turned it into liquid.

'So what's wrong with that?' the lobbies say. The answer: juice isn't even food. When you squeeze a fruit, you turn a food that you crunch and chew into a liquid that you drink.

Again, the principle is the same:

THE MORE YOU TRANSFORM A FOOD, THE MORE WORK THERE IS FOR YOUR PANCREAS.

And this is for a simple reason. Any food you consume must necessarily be broken down into its basic elements to be able to enter the bloodstream.

There are two ways to do this. You can digest it entirely, or you can eat it already transformed, processed, pressed or cooked. The more a food is predigested, the faster it moves through you. And if it's a carbohydrate-rich food, it will be transformed into glucose faster and in higher amounts, which requires the secretion of more insulin.

When you squeeze a fruit – an orange, for example –

take a look at what gets left in the press: all the fibrous web of the pulp has been separated from the juice. That's work that your body would be doing, if you ate fruit the way it comes off the tree.

That's why your job for the last six months of your pregnancy is to replace fruit juice with fresh fruits.

And now's a good time to remind ourselves of what we've been hearing from health organisations for ages now: eat five servings of fruits and vegetables each day.

It's hard to argue with such sound advice. However, some ambiguity hides within it. Grouping the two families of food under the same heading implies that fruits and vegetables are interchangeable. That's not exactly true; and it may lead to some bad decisions.

Everything that you find in fruit – vitamins, minerals and fibres – is found in vegetables as well. But there's a profound difference between the two foods. To summarise it simply: *a fruit is like a sugary vegetable.*

Let's look at a few examples: an average portion of orange or pineapple contains 4 grams of fructose; peach contains 5 grams; watermelon contains 6 grams; grapes contain 8 grams; and pear contains 10 grams.

There are *zero* grams of fructose in spinach, mushrooms, celery, broccoli and lettuce, and 1 to 2 grams in eggplant, asparagus, cabbage and tomatoes. Only carrots and beets have higher amounts.

This fructose presence doesn't cause any problems for people with a strong pancreas; it does become a problem, however, for those whose pancreas is vulnerable. This is the case for people with diabetes, who are advised not to eat a lot of fruit.

A study in the *British Medical Journal* used data on 187,000 people who were monitored over a 24-year period. During that time, 12,000 of them developed type 2 diabetes. In comparing their consumption of whole fruits and fruit juice, they found that replacing three portions of fruit juice with whole fruits reduced the risk of diabetes by 7 per cent. The number rose to 12 per cent for grapefruit; 14 per cent for apples and pears; and 19 per cent for grapes.

It was long believed that fructose, which has higher sweetening power than white sugar, has a lower glycaemic index. It was therefore thought to be a good substitute for sugar.

We now know that fructose is more dangerous for diabetics than glucose, because the liver transforms it more quickly into fat, raising the level of blood triglycerides and helping pave the way for **insulin resistance**.

So, what is dangerous for the worn-out pancreas of someone with diabetes is even more risky for the foetus during these six months on its path to maturity. The risk becomes greater still during months four and five, when the organ is being constructed. Each intake of sugar forces a reflex response during this period. When this response is repeated again and again, it marks the organ and affects its development.

If you're able to buy organic fruit, do so and choose them yourself to try and avoid getting bruised skins (where possible), as this contains even more vitamins and fibres.

Avoid eating fruit by itself, since it consists almost entirely of carbohydrates. Adding just a small amount of fats and proteins can cut fruit's power to penetrate and limit its impact on the pancreas. A single nut and a spoonful of cottage cheese is enough to slow the digestion and absorption of a slice of pineapple.

Always eat your fruit at the end of a meal, and not before it. Why? For the same reason that a Maserati can only drive as fast as a tractor when following one on a highway. It slows down the fruit's digestion.

Also, try to avoid overripe fruit. As fruit matures, its starches are increasingly converted into simple sugars (fructose and glucose).

What's more, all fruits are not equal. Always consider the potential action of a given fruit on your blood sugar, and by extension on your unborn child's pancreas.

Here are some foods ranked according to their glycaemic effect:

- 10: Dates
- 9: Parsnips, lychee (canned, without stones)
- 8: Watermelon, melon, pumpkin and squash
- 7: Dried raisins, sweet potato, dried figs

- 6: Pineapple, apricot, ripe banana, kiwi
- 5: Chestnuts, melon, papaya, mango, lychee, grapes, pineapple
- 4: Plums
- 3: Nectarines, apples, oranges, coconut, plums, fresh figs, peaches, pears, pineapple, tomatoes, passion fruit, mandarins, clementines
- 2: Blackcurrants, cherries, strawberries, raspberries, blackberries, blueberries, goji berries, passion fruit, ground cherries
- 1: Rhubarb, peanuts, pine nuts, almonds, walnuts, cashews, pistachios, hazelnuts, olives

An action plan for eating during these two months

The basic objective of this plan is quite specific: protecting the development of your developing child's pancreas. The aim is NOT to make you lose weight. Nothing in the roadmap for these two months can be considered, in any way, a weight-loss diet.

On the ninety-first day of pregnancy, at the end of the first trimester, the genetic programme will start transforming the undifferentiated stem cells of the child's pancreas into *beta cells* that are capable of producing insulin. And when the majority of these cells have reached maturity, insulin production will finally be fully operational.

Your goal is to do nothing that might disturb the development of the pancreas towards functioning. If you succeed, your child will have much less risk of carrying a vulnerability to excess weight and diabetes. They will have a normal pancreas that is fully capable of mopping up glucose as soon as its concentration becomes toxic – and it will do this for a full lifetime.

Here's an example. If you aren't diabetic, you get up in the morning with a blood glucose level between 0.8 and 1.05 grams/litre. You eat breakfast: toast and jam. Your level rises to 1.3 to 1.5 grams.

Lunch arrives: you eat a sandwich on the go, or some Chinese food – white rice, a few prawns. For dessert: sorbet. The same beta cells are being asked to work, again and again. Mid-afternoon rolls around, and your hunger returns: you indulge in a chocolate bar from the vending machine. More invasive carbs race through your body.

This dietary model is now the norm among urban dwellers. As we work all day and rush about, we don't always have the time or opportunity to cook more traditional meals.

The description may match your own life. But you're an adult. Even if it's not an optimal way to eat, a diet like this won't affect you much for years to come.

The same is *not* true for the beta cells in the pancreas of a foetus entering the fourth month of pregnancy. The genetic programme that orchestrates the development of the pancreas doesn't plan for such an avalanche of glucose in a single day at such an early age. It's like someone taking their first sailing lesson, suddenly confronting a massive ocean storm.

These first incipient cells are barely capable of secreting, and yet they're forced to start working to produce insulin very early. The task that exceeds their abilities. If this maternal diet, for which the genetic programme does not plan, is maintained over the course of these two months, the infant's pancreas will not thrive. Having to exert itself too early and intensely, it will grow to an abnormal size, secrete too much insulin, produce excess weight and end up becoming exhausted from the stress.

This excessive glucose exposure isn't a problem for pancreatic cells alone. It has effects on all the body's cells that use glucose as fuel: for instance, the cells of the liver, and the muscles, which not only consume glucose but also store it as glycogen. Being put to work too early and with too much demand, these cells will lose their sensitivity to insulin earlier than normal, becoming insulin resistant.

It should be clear now why I place so much importance on your diet over these two months. In these sixty days, you alone can decide the outcome for an organ that will play such a vital role in your child's life.

Over the course of these two months, I'm asking you to *eat for two*. It's an expression you've heard before, but I don't mean you should eat twice as much as usual. Instead, you should be *eating to nourish two different individuals via one mouth*.

Over the two months I'm talking about here, your diet and that of your unborn child must be aligned and controlled in terms of one variable: its processed sugar content.

You can tolerate processed sugar; your child can't.

To make this diet clearer to you and ensure you feel good about adopting it, let's consider the general carbohydrate family. We can divide carbohydrates into three categories based on how harmful they are to the infant's pancreas.

- One: the most invasive and penetrating foods. These you should *eliminate entirely*.
- Two: foods that are rich in carbohydrates but haven't been extensively transformed. These you should *limit* in your diet.
- Three: carbohydrate-based once again, but in a natural state, with little tampering (or processing) involved. *Consume them at your discretion.*

List I: High-carbohydrate foods to ELIMINATE during these two months

These are ranked in descending order according to their invasive effect on the development of the foetal pancreas.

- **Beer.** This is probably the food that is *least* tolerated by an adult pancreas, and infinitely less tolerated by a pancreas that is going through differentiation. Because it's an alcoholic beverage, your doctor has probably prohibited it anyway.
- **Potatoes**
  - **Instant potato flakes.** In its industrially processed form, this hyper-processed food comes in a pretty

package that makes it practical and easy to prepare. It's also one of the most quickly absorbed solid foods, and therefore extremely aggressive towards the pancreas.

- **Boiled and peeled potatoes**
- **Baked potatoes**
- **French fries**
- **Chips**
- **Potato gnocchi**

- Bread
  - **Gluten-free white bread.** You may be surprised to hear me go against the raging gluten-free trend. To be clear, this recommendation only concerns pregnancy – specifically, those two crucial months. If you don't have a gluten intolerance, neither you nor your child has any reason to fear gluten. Gluten, like protein, slows down the digestion and assimilation of sugars contained in wheat flour. Also, about 10 per cent of the proteins have been eliminated from gluten-free bread; it automatically contains more carbohydrates.
  - **Rusks of pure white flour.** Here, the disadvantages of white flour are reinforced by the fact that the rusks, as their name indicates, are cooked twice, which further sharpens the penetration power of the flour.
  - **Any ultra-white bread.** The crust of a bread is a bit more resistant to digestion than the rest of the loaf. For this reason, producers – as usual, doing anything possible to open the door wide for carbohydrates –

have gone so far as to create a crustless loaf of bread, sliced for sandwiches. *Why?*

- **French bread.** In France, the baguette is pretty much a sacred tradition; and French bread is enjoyed around the world. Remember, we're only talking about two months here.

- **Corn flakes.** We took a careful look at the many rounds of industrial transformation forced on to corn to make it more penetrating. Corn flakes are the processed food par excellence; they're transformed to make them visually appealing and gives them a pleasant consistency, at the cost of their nutritional value. I'm convinced that this food, invented in the United States, has played a role in causing the American obesity epidemic. **Its responsibility is all the greater in that the product targets children, marketed as a breakfast meal. With this combination of age group and time of day, the danger from carbohydrates is very high.**

Corn flakes can contribute to your vitality and balance. Nevertheless, among the large family of corn flakes, not all are as aggressive and diabetogenic. Those that are the least are those that contain the most protein and fat. As paradoxical as it may seem, the fact that corn flakes contain chocolate reduces their glycaemic index and their impact on the foetal pancreas. Be wary of certain corn flakes that are presented as diet products, or even slimming. Such products would be almost funny if the advertisement did not make them appear credible.

Cornflour. Some cooks use small amounts to thicken sauces; the risk then isn't very high. Still, better to wait until the end of the crucial two months; all the better for the pancreas that's budding within your foetus.

- **Aggressive kinds of rice**
  - **Fast-cooking rice.** To save time for consumers, rice producers precook rice. This action is essentially physical predigestion; it elevates the penetrating power of the rice's carbohydrates.
  - **Sticky rice.** Usually found in Chinese cooking. If you have the option to choose between sticky or normal rice during the crucial two months, opt for normal. (You'll find it under the second category of carbohydrates.)
  - **Puffed rice.** Rice whose husk has been removed with a combination of strong pressure and water vapour. That makes it fun, easy to eat, and up to three times the volume of the original grain. However, it is digested much faster and has a powerful penetrative power.

    In India, where many still suffer from hunger, puffed rice (pori) is used as a religious offering. Here, as elsewhere, dietary traditions and religion have adapted in tandem to respond to the needs of the public. The religious use of puffed rice led Indians to consume it themselves – the food became a staple in shortage areas.

    Turning rice into puffed rice makes it more

profitable, and makes it advantageous for survival. It doesn't increase the calorie count, but it makes it flood into the blood more quickly and in greater quantities. Then more insulin is needed to transform these sugars into fat. What was a blessing for malnourished Indians has turned into a problem for those who live in a culture of abundance where food has been extensively industrialised.

- **Rice cakes.** The same things are true as for puffed rice. However, they're often organic and presented as health food – a balanced snack. The opposite is true. Marketers tell you that their light weight (around eight grams) is linked to *your* light weight (present or future). And always remember that organic doesn't mean a low glycaemic risk. A food can be grown under the best, pesticide-free conditions and still be diabetogenic.

- **Biscuits made with white flour.** These biscuits should be avoided entirely during the sensitive two months. However, this does not mean you have to avoid all biscuits.

Let's approach it in clear and concrete terms. Manufacturers are required to list the nutritional value, often for 100 grams of a product. If you really want to estimate the carbohydrate risk of a food – a risk to the development of your child's pancreas – you need to understand what this carbohydrate amount *means*.

The carbohydrate measurement you see for a biscuit is

mainly based on sugar and the cereal it contains. Because we know that white flour has an even higher glycaemic index than sugar, these two ingredients will race against each other to enter the blood. As shocking as it may seem, the winner will be white flour.

If you're neither diabetic nor overweight, you can tolerate this type of biscuit for years. If you are diabetic, eating them creates pressure on your pancreas that should be avoided. But if you're pregnant, the pressure is exerted on a fragile developing pancreas. If the exposure is regular, there's a risk of weakening this organ and creating a permanent vulnerability.

Biscuits are one of the snack industry's main products today. If you're going to buy them, it's important that you know how to choose them properly – today for your child's sake, tomorrow for your own. For this you only need to consider three criteria: the carbohydrate level, the white sugar level and the type of grain used.

If it's wheat, the flour used will be white and will be absorbed ultra-quickly in your body. If the flour is whole-wheat, it will consist of white flour to which a token amount of wheat bran has been added. The mixture separates in the stomach to become white flour again. If, however, the flour is whole-grain wheat or rye, the invasive power is truly slower.

The slowest grain is oat bran, with a glycaemic index of 15. That's about five times slower than white flour, which is 80.

Be very careful when you read the packaging on biscuits. Don't rely on manufacturers' claims that a food product is 'part of a balanced diet'. Trust only the list of ingredients and the carbohydrate levels on the nutritional label. These two facts mean a lot more than any other kind of health claim.

When you're past your pregnancy, I suggest you keep the habit of going by these three criteria – for yourself and for your family.

If a serving of a food has more than 50 grams of carbohydrates, coming from processed white flour or processed white sugar, you're putting strain on your pancreas. And even if it's not a foetal pancreas, it's so easy to switch to biscuits made with a whole-grain flour, which is denser, more consistent and actually tastes of the earth. Unfortunately, it's hard to find in supermarkets.

- **White sugar or sucrose.** As you can see, sugar is far from the top of the list. Note that the colour – brown, for instance – makes no difference for its nutritional value. Remember: sugar is a nutritional void.

- **All sweets, hard or soft.** Sweets are primarily made of sugar. But whereas we normally add spoonfuls of sugar to other foods, sweets have added colour and flavouring, inviting one and all to indulge.

- **Sugary soft drinks.** This type of beverage consists mainly of two things: water and sugar. More than half have more than 100 grams of sugar per litre: that's the equivalent of twenty sugar cubes. You might remember New York City mayor Michael Bloomberg imposing a ban on soft drink cups over half a litre in volume a few years ago. Bloomberg was actually aware of my work fighting invasive sugars and asked for my support for his project. It was a happy day for both of us when the city's health department authorised the ban. Unfortunately, the American Beverage Association succeeded in pressuring the federal government to reject the measure.

- **Sugary sorbets.** They consist of fruit juices to which sugar and water are added. During these two months, resolutely set aside the sorbet and avoid the ice if possible.
- **Noodles made from soft wheat** should be left on grocery store shelves until your baby's pancreas is more mature. It's not much to ask. Other kinds of pasta are easy to find: spaghetti, cooked *al dente*, for example.
- **Dates** are probably the most sugary fruit that has ever existed. Dates and raisins are the only dried fruits that you should really avoid altogether during those two months.

List II: High-carbohydrate foods to AVOID during the crucial two months

The first list contained foods that you should **eliminate** because they are too aggressive for your unborn child. This list contains foods you should **avoid altogether**.

This project is valuable enough that it is worth taking any steps we can to prevent frustration.

Clearly, each pregnancy is unique. You may therefore be asking yourself if the details of this plan are equally valid for all pregnancies.

When it comes to the first list, the answer is unequivocally *yes*. No matter your weight, your heredity, your level of physical activity, these foods are *distinctly* at odds with the design of the human body. We think of them as edible, but they undermine our biological foundation.

Why? Simply because we were not designed to consume them. Our organs are not capable of handling them for any significant length of time.

When it comes to an adult's pancreas, think again of the metaphor of a lock with the wrong key. If you force it, the lock may open for a certain number of times, creaking and straining; but each time, it will require more effort, until finally it jams.

And this comparison applies only to the pancreas of an adult today. You may think your pancreas is running smoothly, but many of us have a pancreas that's becoming weaker and more damaged each day.

The number of diabetics doubled in France in one generation. And the progression is identical for obesity.

But as I have emphasised: this plan is not for *your* pancreas, but for that of the child you're carrying.

When you came into this world – probably at least twenty-five years ago, in another generation's time – your mother almost certainly didn't have access to the same supermarket chains that you do.

She herself was probably carried, birthed and raised in a world where bread was ubiquitous, as it is now; but it was made of an entirely different kind of flour. She lived in a world where mothers prepared their own biscuits, where corn flakes, puffed rice, white sandwich bread, fast-cooking rice and maybe even Coca-Cola were nowhere to be found; where putting sugary ketchup on meat would be thought of as bizarre.

Today, as I write this book and offer you a plan to follow, what matters to me most of all is the pancreas belonging to that little boy or girl you're preparing to bring into the world. It's a pancreas that is part of the next generation, of which your child will be part.

This little lock must be forged in a calm environment, free from shocks and with care for its function.

For the second carbohydrate list, what matters most is the notion of quantity. If you're a perfectionist and you're able to totally avoid the products it contains, I commend you – I think that's the best strategy. But if you and your doctor think you can consume those foods occasionally, be very sure to limit the quantity.

- **Standard white rice**, the kind you get in Chinese or Japanese restaurants. If you can't avoid it, try to leave some at the bottom of the bowl. And remember to avoid sticky rice, which is white but more invasive; it's on the list of **foods to eliminate**.
- **Finely ground white couscous.** Couscous comes in three

sizes: large, medium and small. The smallest version is the one to avoid. Couscous is further proof of the fact that the more you physically or chemically process a food, the less work is required during digestion, the less resistance the food meets and the more quickly it arrives in the blood.

The large-size couscous – essentially Moroccan Berber couscous – is almost impossible to find, and takes a few minutes more to cook. If you like a grainy consistency, you'll love this kind.

Whatever the size, avoid cooking this grain for long: this accelerates the transformation of carbohydrates into glucose.

- **Ordinary semolina.** For these two months, choose whole-grain semolina.
- **Bread with 30 per cent rye.** Specifically, this is bread *with* rye, containing 30 per cent of that ingredient, and not *rye bread,* which has about 60 per cent rye. The difference between the two kinds is that the 30 per cent difference usually consists of white flour.
- **Canned corn.** The kernels stripped from the ear have aged in the can and are steeped in liquid; they're predigested, robbing you of the opportunity to do the digesting.
- **Ice cream.** You'll notice that I made a distinction between ice cream, which is to be avoided, and sorbet, which is to be eliminated. That's because ice cream, while having more calories, contains milk, cream or eggs, which slow down carbohydrate absorption.

This distinction should highlight the fact that calories matter less than the categories they belong to. It might seem like splitting hairs, but it's one of the main reasons the fight against excess weight and diabetes is so often thwarted.

For a long time now, a concerted effort has been made to hide the dangers of invasive carbohydrates. One of the most effective tactics is to claim that:

'One calorie = one calorie' and that 'All calories are equal'.

This apparently simple, logical idea belies a monstrous deception, conscious or otherwise. The unit of measurement casts a veil over *what it is* we're measuring. Think of it like this: if 1 gram really equals 1 gram, a gram of cyanide is equal to a gram of baking soda.

The same goes for the popular and longstanding myth that proteins are harmful to the kidney. This is simply a smokescreen to make us forget that it's sugar, not proteins that are responsible for damaging the kidneys.

Similarly, Coca-Cola recently focused its marketing on physical activity, skilfully leading us to think that, if you increase your level of physical activity, you can keep drinking sugary fizzy drinks.

- **Ripe bananas.** Bananas are already one of the most high-glycaemic fruits. But as they ripen, the starch chains transform into infinitely more invasive glucose: that means their glycaemic index level rises even higher. The same phenomenon takes place when you cook a banana, and for the same reasons.

- **Cooked beans.** If you really love beans and the legume is in season, why not try them raw, young and tender, without the shell? In this form, you can indulge to your heart's desire.

- **Buckwheat flour.** Aside from its high amounts of carbohydrates (72 g/100 g), buckwheat is allergenic. According to Dr Castelain-Hacquet, head of allergology at France's Saint-Vincent de Paul Hospital: 'There were 14 cases of severe anaphylaxis to buckwheat since 2010, including five in 2014 – the last one took place on Tuesday. All the patients treated received first aid kit containing adrenalin.' [25] If you love buckwheat pancakes, wait until your pregnancy is over.

- **Canned pineapple.** Pineapple is a fruit that's high on the glycaemic index, and eating it canned in syrup bumps it even higher. You may have heard that the fruit contains bromelain, a magic enzyme that melts cellulite. This is a myth. This enzyme facilitates the digestion of proteins, but not fats, and especially not cellulite.

- **Well-cooked white spaghetti.** In the third list, below, you'll see that spaghetti cooked *al dente* is tolerable, but the same pasta cooked for longer is not, for the small developing pancreas. I'll risk becoming repetitive here and say it again: the more extensively a food is processed,

---

[25] *Le Monde: Science and Technology*, 28 April 2012.

the faster you will absorb it, and the more it will raise your own and your unborn child's pancreas. Cooking is part of that transformation. If a diabetic could eat raw potatoes, there would be no reason to prohibit them; but in their ready-to-use flaked form, it would be dangerous.

- **Regular ketchup.** Ketchup is a mixture of tomatoes, vinegar and sugar. Its carbohydrate level is 26 g/100. A fresh tomato contains only 3.9 grams, and mustard has 5 grams. Try making your own ketchup. If you have time, start with fresh tomatoes – if not, use tomato paste.

- **Bulgur, well cooked.** The same is true of pasta made from hard wheat. Excessive cooking heightens its invasive power.

- **Long-grain brown rice and red Thai rice.** These are less invasive than white rice, but you should still avoid them during that short but crucial period for your child's developing pancreas.

- **Nutella.** You'll probably be surprised to find Nutella in the category of foods that are to be avoided and not eliminated outright. The reason for this is that the fat content that accompanies the sugar slows its progression.

- **Whole-wheat bread.** This too is to be avoided: the word 'whole' is misleading. All it means is that wheat has been added to white flour. Beer poured into a wine glass is still beer.

- **Whole-wheat pasta.** To be avoided for the crucial two months. On the list below, you'll see that you can eat whole-grain pasta, cooked *al dente*.

- **Sweet potato.** It's better than regular potato, but still, wait for two months.
- **Pre-packaged pizza**, because of the flour. Wait till the crucial two months are over, then make your own pizza with whole-grain flour – and don't forget a spoonful of oil to slow down the 'sugars'.
- **Basmati rice (long grain).** If you love the flavour of basmati, you'll find it on the list below, but in a whole-grain version.
- **Honey** should really be avoided during those two months. Even though it's a natural product, it's adapted for bees, not humans, and especially not for a developing foetus. Honey is a near-pure mixture of fructose and glucose.
- **Canned lychee** is to be avoided – canned only, though.
- **Waffles.** Avoid shop-bought waffles: they're made mainly with white flour. But if you want to take the time to prepare whole-grain or oat bran flour yourself, that's an option.

List III: Foods tolerated in moderate quantities

The third list doesn't contain things to eliminate or even to avoid. These are things you can consume. But that doesn't mean you should overdo it. Don't forget what you learned in Chapter 8: how to calculate the glycaemic load. The point isn't for you to be an expert in the nutritional information that diabetics need to know. The main thing *you* need to know is that, when it comes to carbohydrates, quality is as important as quantity.

Thus, this third list contains foods that you can eat, but not in excessive portions. Warning: while these foods have an acceptable quantity of 'sugars', they can still accumulate and reach unacceptable levels very quickly.

- **Wild rice.** This would be your best option for rice – if it were actually rice. Wild rice is an aquatic plant that's hard to find. Overcooking it can make it unappealing. The best solution is to let it soak in water for a few hours or overnight, before cooking.
- **Whole-grain basmati rice.** Basmati + whole grain = your open door. But even though it's Indian in origin, eat it Italian style: *al dente*.
- **Tabbouleh.** Lebanese style, with lots of parsley, mint, onions and tomatoes mixed in with the bulgur.
- **Bulgur.** A type of cracked wheat that's shelled and precooked.
- **Vegetable wheat.** A little different from bulgur, it differs in the fact that it is whole and not crushed.
- **Shop-bought tomato sauce.** It does contain sugar, but in reasonable amounts. If you want to, you can find sugar-free sauces as well.
- **Pumpernickel.** A heavy German bread rich in fibres and little-processed grains. If you don't have weight problems, try it with crushed avocado.
- **Rye bread (60 per cent rye).** Not *with rye* but *rye* – an important distinction.
- **Whole-grain couscous**

- **Whole-grain kamut and kamut bread.** A species of wheat whose grains are quite a bit bigger and harder than ordinary wheat, which gives it a more resistant husk; slower to break down, it is lower on the glycaemic index. Unfortunately, you may only be able to find it in health-food stores.
- **Whole-grain wheat flour.** Stone-ground flour that is little sifted; it isn't stripped of its bran, germ or starch.
- **Whole-grain spaghetti, cooked *al dente*.** Add some butter and Parmesan to slow the absorption of carbohydrates.
- **Sugar-free whole-grain breadsticks.** Don't forget that these tolerated foods add up in combination.
- **100 per cent whole-grain sourdough**
- **Whole-grain pasta, cooked *al dente***
- **Raw cider.** To give you some idea:
  - 15 cl of raw cider = 1 cube of sugar
  - 15 cl of sweet cider = 2 cubes of sugar
  - 10 cl of Madeira wine = 2 cubes of sugar
  - 25 cl of beer = 2.5 cubes of sugar
  - 10 cl of Muscat dessert wine = 4 sugars
- **Coconut milk.** A jewel for cooks who want to give their dishes an exotic touch and a richer flavour. It's a main ingredient in Thai food and part of the reason the cuisine is so popular today. For those who might be tempted to eat too much of it, you can cut the amount and mix with equal parts of coconut water. It's also a great milk replacement for those who are lactose intolerant.
- **Agave syrup and coconut sugar.** To avoid sweeteners

totally devoid of carbohydrates, these two natural sweeteners are good substitutes with low glycaemic levels.

• **Pumpkin and squash.** Both are great to eat in soups during the crucial two months.

List IV: Carbohydrates to eat freely

The fourth list contains foods that are high in carbohydrates but whose molecular configuration makes them slower to digest and absorb, and therefore less disturbing for your baby's development. As you will see, this book's enemy isn't carbohydrates but rather their penetrating power.

The tolerated foods mentioned above cover the vast majority of your pregnancy needs – as well as your gustatory pleasure – but without placing violent demands on the pancreas of the beloved little passenger in your womb.

As you select and prepare your food, don't forget that everything you put in your mouth will be shared with them.

Remember that all the carbohydrates you ingest become glucose; glucose generates insulin; and insulin is the cause of the problems we're concerned with.

So if you eat a club sandwich on white bread, or a plate of risotto with a beer, massive amounts of glucose will flood your blood and that of your child. This unexpected concentration of glucose requires the foetus to produce insulin but also to create new factories to produce that insulin: endocrine beta cells.

Our objective during this period is to help you get the

carbohydrates you need, but bit by bit, rather than in avalanche form – in a slow and regulated way, to avoid the brutal spike in blood sugar and the equally violent response of your pancreas, with its massive release of insulin. Be like a mouse walking quietly in front of a sleeping cat, trying not to wake it. During those two months, choose 'silent' foods.

It's a colourful metaphor, but the point is essential. Consider, too, the alternative tale, based on the intake of dangerous foods: large, noisy rats making a colossal racket, abruptly wakening a sleeping cat, which reflexively attacks, using all the weapons at its disposal.

So what are these silent carbohydrates? That's the subject of our fourth list: foods you can eat normally, without worrying.

- **Peas and chickpeas.** These are the champions of slow carbohydrates. While you should avoid or eliminate certain very invasive starchy or floury foods, these, prepared properly, can make great replacements.
- **Kidney beans, black beans, yellow or brown lentils.** These are food powerhouses: dense, filling, rich in fibre and high in nutritional value.
- **Stew and homemade sauerkraut**: avoid canned foods.
- **Nectarines.** Try not to have more than three portions of fruit per day during the two crucial months.
- **Rye crispbreads** made up of 24 per cent fibre.
- **Apples, oranges, pears, grapefruit, currants, cherries,**

strawberries, raspberries. Remember: three portions a day will suffice.

- **Fresh tomatoes**
- **Tomato juice.** Tomatoes have high nutritional value, and their lycopene content helps prevent certain cancers.
- **Sugar-free tomato sauce**, shop-bought or homemade.
- **Quinoa.** A trendy food that's rich in proteins (16 to 18 per cent) and iron, high in biological value and free of gluten. The grain has a caviar-like texture that bursts when you bite it, with a slight hazelnut flavour. It's great in savoury and sweet dishes alike.
- **Yogurt and white cream cheese/cottage cheese** – sugar-free, but not necessarily light.
- **Sugar-free diet chocolate bar**, if you feel the need.
- **Green beans**
- **Artichokes**
- **Dark chocolate, 70 per cent or higher.** In moderation, if your doctor is monitoring your weight. The sugar in the chocolate is slowed by the accompanying fat.

List V: Recommended carbohydrates

The last list contains virtuous foods: those that you're not only permitted but actually encouraged to eat – especially if you have an active lifestyle.

Neuroscientists know that, at every level on the animal scale, habit is a kind of **biological impulse that promotes individual safety and survival**. Any behaviour that is repeated and doesn't lead to harm is recognised as safe and is admitted. But if a behaviour proves more than merely safe and ends up gratifying and soothing, it is installed in our brain circuitry as a desirable habit.

Pregnancy is generally one of the most rewarding events in a woman's life. The habits that develop during that time take deeper roots than most. So, to make your pregnancy as safe as possible, take up the habit of reducing your consumption of invasive carbohydrates. It'll be that much easier to keep the habit going after you give birth – especially if you have weight problems or a family history of diabetes, cardiovascular disease or cancer.

Here are the very beneficial foods you can eat on a daily basis:

- **All green vegetables**, particularly all kinds of cabbage, zucchini, mushrooms, any type of lettuce, cucumber, radishes, leeks, spinach, peppers, fennel, endives, tomatoes and eggplant
- **Lemon, strawberries and raspberries**
- **Palm heart**
- **Snow peas**
- **Oilseeds, including nuts, hazelnuts, almonds, pine nuts, avocados and olives**
- **Rhubarb** is tart and rich in fibres and extremely low in carbohydrates. Try making compote: fresh-tasting and rich in fibre. The icing on the cake is that rhubarb is rich in antioxidant polyphenols, and it was recently

discovered to contain parietin, a pigment that can inhibit the growth of cancerous tumours.

- **Lupin flour** which you can use as an addition if you are preparing pastry. Its glycaemic index is as low as that of oat bran.

- **Cocoa with 1 per cent fat.** In recent years, cacao has been available with lower and lower amounts of fat: first 21 per cent, then 11 per cent, and finally 1 per cent. Try the latter. It's great for baking, and gives you that slightly euphoric chocolate feeling so many of us love.

- **And finally, oat bran**, a food I truly love. Its primary virtue is that it can replace flour perfectly for almost any usage, without compromising its incredible glycaemic index level. It's extremely useful to keep the following in mind:

  - **Glucose has a glycaemic index of 100** (think about it as the maximum speed of a car)

  - And **white sugar and sucrose have a glycaemic index of 70**

  - **And today's white flour has a glycaemic index of 80**

  - **The glycaemic index of oat bran is 15.**

These are the elements you should respect for those two crucial months – those sixty days that are so important for the future of your pregnancy.

As you can see, the recommendations are clear, simple and easy to follow.

During these essential two months, you can eat anything

that is healthy and beneficial. You won't be missing anything you need, and you won't be consuming processed invasive carbohydrates, which today we know are partly responsible for the global epidemic in excess weight and diabetes.

For the most part, these are industrially processed foods that have been altered and made artificial through multiple physical and chemical processing. These alterations are intended to transform them into 'convenient' merchandise: cheap, enticing and easy to consume. But the processing they undergo also makes you digest and absorb them faster, which means a massive secretion of insulin. The refining of their carbohydrates also transforms them into addictive substances that work on the brain's reward and dependence circuits.

These foods are **dangerous** for adults in the medium term, if they consume them regularly and with abandon. And if they're dangerous for adults, they're even more so for a developing baby – especially during those two months when the power to synthesise insulin is starting to form.

The last four months of your pregnancy: The sixth, seventh, eighth and ninth month.

If you've reached the third period of your pregnancy and you've followed the guidelines for the fourth and fifth months, you've successfully navigated that critical period and you're no longer in the eye of the hurricane.

But be careful: it's not all over.

At the end of the first trimester, the initial buds of your

child's pancreas have joined, and the organ has taken its rightful position in the abdomen.

During the following two months, the fourth and fifth months, the differentiated beta cells within the islets of Langerhans have multiplied and started secreting their first drops of insulin.

This miniature pancreas is now developed. It has started to function: it knows how to recognise glucose and has the means to respond to variations of concentration in the blood.

Why is the danger weighing on your child's pancreas reduced in the last two months? Because during this phase of cell proliferation, the process can be sent into overdrive due to an overly glycaemic diet.

Starting from the sixth month, the cells of the pancreas (now a properly formed organ) multiply less, but grow larger. The little pancreas follows their development, becoming larger and producing more and more insulin until birth.

During the same period, the mother's body naturally goes through a period of insulin resistance. This helps her to gain weight, improving her chances of carrying the pregnancy to term. The process is still inscribed in our genetic score. However, the danger today is actually abundance, rather than lack; that means we need to be very aware of this natural tendency. The intensity of the insulin resistance varies according to maternal body weight before pregnancy, the number of previous pregnancies and family history of excess weight or diabetes.

In the last trimester, all your body's cells, especially those of the liver and muscles, will lose some of their sensitivity to insulin. That means you need more insulin to neutralise and suppress the same quantity of glucose. If your diet remains too rich in invasive carbohydrates, you therefore run the risk of damaging your pancreas. It's usually in the dietary and hormonal context of the third semester that weight gain starts to get out of control and the risk of gestational diabetes increases.

The dietary guidelines intended to protect the foetus during this last phase of pregnancy will also benefit you if you're at risk of gestational diabetes. Today there's some debate about increasing monitoring for gestational diabetes, especially for at-risk women. Risk level is related to the presence of excess weight, a family history of diabetes and previously having given birth to a large baby. Gestational diabetes may be unpreventable in some cases. If it does appear, reducing 'sugars' is not enough, and insulin is needed.

That means that limiting invasive diabetogenic sugars in order to protect the foetus can also benefit the mother: both pancreases face the same threat.

To summarise: at the beginning of the sixth month, you'll be ending the period of your pregnancy when the risk of establishing a vulnerability in your unborn child's pancreas is highest.

If you have followed the advice in this book over the two crucial months and limited the amount of 'invasive sugars' you consume, the little pancreas has been developing according to the genetic programme of our species.

But if you haven't been convinced and you've abused the foods that hinder that organ's development, there's a significant risk that your child has developed a pancreas with an overabundance of cells that secrete too much insulin, and has developed a vulnerability that may last a lifetime.

At this point, while the risk related to the multiplication of pancreatic cells has lessened, it has not disappeared. Even if the danger has waned, you should continue to watch your diet carefully. The plan offered to you here aims to help avoid excessive insulin production. Too many high-glycaemic foods means too much insulin will be inscribed in the biological memory of the foetus too early. The result is an expected increase in the risk of insulin resistance.

In practice, during the last four months of pregnancy, it's wise to stick to the Five Basic Steps (page 193). These principles are enough to constitute a solid line of defence for the foetal pancreas.

But these rules go beyond protecting your child. With practice, they can become dietary reflexes that will protect you from an artificial and diabetogenic diet that we've come to think of as normal – and which is anything but normal. Its recent invasion directly correlates with the global epidemic in excess weight, obesity and diabetes.

Therefore, it's a good idea to continue the diet past your pregnancy, to integrate it into your daily life and to share it with the people you care about. Foods as common as corn flakes, instant potatoes, sugary fizzy drinks and white bread are not foods for humans. Why? Because we have neither the organs nor the physiologies that can assimilate them safely.

But let's return to the subject of your child. Along with the Five Basic Steps, it's a good idea to continue avoiding foods that require your pancreas to secrete too much insulin. The more you're tempted to consume, the bigger your child will get and the higher their birth weight will be.

During the two previous months, all you're asked to do is eliminate nineteen foods and avoid twenty-four.

For the last four months, you no longer need to radically cut out any foods – only to generally avoid the ones in the following list. 'Avoid' means do what you can to not consume them, and, above all, don't abuse them. This limitation will protect your child's health for the rest of their life. And if you keep going in that general direction, if the lesson leaves its mark on you, it will protect your own health too.

I kept the number of processed foods to avoid at nineteen so that implementing the plan will be painless. But I ask that you follow it rigorously and attentively. None of the foods is useful to you; they're anything but indispensable. The human species has done without them for 199,950 of its 200,000 years of existence – you are fully capable of doing the same. You'll even enjoy it.

YOUR DAILY DIET

The nineteen foods below are to be eliminated – not avoided. The difference in terminology corresponds to a significant difference in risk.

The nineteen foods to avoid:

1) Beer
2) Instant potato flakes
3) Peeled boiled potatoes or baked potatoes
4) Fries and chips
5) Gluten-free white bread
6) Pure white flour
7) White sandwich bread
8) French bread
9) Corn flakes
10) Cornflour
11) Fast-cooking rice and sticky rice
12) Puffed rice and rice cakes
13) Biscuits made with white flour
14) White sugar (sucrose)
15) Sweets, hard and soft
16) Sugary fizzy drinks
17) Sweet sorbets
18) Soft wheat noodles
19) Dates and raisins

How to deal with other
high-carbohydrate foods

The risk for these foods is lower, but it still exists. As you can see, the list includes foods like white rice, couscous, corn, well-cooked pasta – all part of the family of starchy foods.

Today's recommendations tell us to eat starches regularly: one or two servings a day. These guidelines may present no problem for those who have no problem limiting their portions and who therefore have no weight problems or diabetes. But for others – nearly half of adults today – it's not so easy.

In the 1950s, the United Nations' Food and Agriculture Organization recommended that carbohydrates make up 55 per cent of our daily caloric intake.

Today, sixty-five years later (and despite the eradication of physical activity), the same rate of 55 per cent holds – its origin long forgotten.

This isn't the moment for a political debate. The health of your unborn child, however, is another matter. This developing child doesn't belong to our time, and especially not to our culture. It exists in a matrix that's directly connected to our origins. To put it simply, until the moment this child-to-be is born, nothing distinguishes it biologically from a primitive hunter-gatherer. And those laws of nature tell us that the child's body, organs and physiology have no basis to accept a starch-filled diet without suffering side effects.

If, when you're not pregnant, you regularly eat a lot of starchy foods and you don't gain weight, you're one of the lucky few. But if you are pregnant, learn how to distinguish between carbohydrates for the last four months. I've classified them into four groups: those to eliminate, those to avoid, those to limit, and those that you're free to eat and share with others.

As you navigate the last four months, you can lower your level of vigilance by one level.

- The list of foods to ELIMINATE becomes foods to AVOID
- Foods to AVOID can now be LIMITED
- And the other three categories are now TO BE EATEN FREELY.

1) High-carbohydrate foods to AVOID

- Standard white rice. I recommend asking specifically for whole-grain rice if you go to a restaurant. Reminder: no sticky rice.
- Fine white couscous. Switch to medium grain, and cook it as little as possible.
- Ordinary semolina. For these four months, use whole-grain semolina.
- Switch from bread with rye (30 per cent) to rye bread (60 per cent).
- Canned corn, in kernels. Switch to grilled corn on the cob.
- Ice cream (only eat it if you can't refuse).

- No ripe bananas. Switch to yellow bananas with no marks.
- Cooked beans. Switch to fresh beans, eaten fresh.
- Buckwheat flour: avoid due to allergy risk.
- Canned pineapple: eat fresh.
- Switch from well-cooked white spaghetti to whole-grain spaghetti, *al dente*.
- Regular ketchup
- Bulgur, whole-grain brown rice and red Thai rice should be avoided, or eaten only in small quantities.
- Nutella (for a while), although you can indulge in small amounts of dark chocolate.
- Whole-wheat bread. Switch to whole-grain.
- Whole-wheat pasta: look for whole-grain instead.
- Sweet potato: eat only occasionally.
- Honey: limit as much as possible.
- Canned lychee: opt for fresh.
- Homemade waffles: eliminate store-bought waffles.

2) Carbohydrate foods to consume FREELY

- Wild rice
- Whole-grain basmati rice (*al dente*)
- Tabouleh
- Bulgur
- Durum wheat
- Shop-bought tomato sauce (sugar-free can be found, but it may contain some sugar)
- Pumpernickel
- Whole-grain couscous

- Whole-grain kamut flour and kamut bread
- Whole-wheat flour
- Whole-grain spaghetti *al dente*
- Whole-grain breadsticks (sugar-free)
- 100 per cent whole-grain sourdough
- Whole-grain pasta *al dente*
- Coconut milk
- Pumpkin and squash
- Peas and chickpeas
- Kidney beans, black beans, yellow and brown lentils
- Homemade sauerkraut
- Rye crispbreads
- Nectarines, apples, pears, grapefruit, currants, cherries, strawberries, raspberries – try not to exceed three portions of fruits per day
- Fresh tomatoes, tomato juice, sugar-free tomato sauce
- Quinoa
- Yogurt and white Cheddar – not necessarily light, but sugar-free
- Sugar-free diet chocolate bars, if you feel the urge
- Artichokes

3) Recommended carbohydrate foods

Here are the everyday foods that are very beneficial.

- All green vegetables, particularly mushrooms, all types of cabbage, zucchini, all types of lettuce, cucumbers, radishes, leeks, spinach, green beans

- Peppers, fennel, endives, tomatoes and eggplant
- Lemons, strawberries and raspberries
- Palm hearts
- Snow peas
- Coco beans
- Oilseeds: nuts, hazelnuts, almonds, pine nuts, avocados, olives
- Rhubarb
- Lupin flour (see also page 227)
- Cocoa with 1 per cent fat
- Oat bran

Moving on together

As you come to the end of this book, I hope you have been persuaded to follow the plan for the last six months of your pregnancy.

If you're starting a pregnancy and you haven't been convinced, you still have three months to reflect – three months in which your child's pancreas does not yet exist. Consider carefully: a diet low in industrially processed foods is simply a return to the diet your grandmother had when she was carrying your mother.

So much evidence exists today on how harmful invasive sugars are for an adult human that it's easy to ignore the effect it can have on the little being inside you.

On the other hand, if you've decided to follow the plan, then nothing could make me happier. And in that case, I'd like to ask for your help in taking the plan further.

How? Merely by keeping a simple journal of your diet for the six months of the plan.

There are two reasons I'm asking you to do this.

One, it will be a way to collect and keep information on your consumption of carbohydrates over the six months of your pregnancy. It can then be analysed in combination with all the other journals, and used to fight weight and health problems in the children born of these pregnancies. The more readers who send in their results, the more meaningful the results will be.

Today we know that the obesity and diabetes epidemic manifests very early on. One of the first warning signs is birth weight. Even more important is the weight of the infant at six months, and more still the weight at two years.

Each day, note down the foods you've consumed to show if you've eaten a little, a moderate amount or a lot, so the results can be tabulated. It only takes a few seconds.

At the end of your pregnancy, note down the gender, weight and birthday of your child. And if you're willing, also monitor your child's weight at six months, one year and two years. (You can also do this online, via my free website www.baby6months.com.)

This should all help prove (or disprove) the fundamental point that is the basis for this whole project.

And if the basis of this book is proven correct – and I'm certain it will be – imagine the satisfaction of knowing how much you've done for your child's health and future.

And imagine my satisfaction at having helped you get there.

If you follow the plan in this book, I invite you to write to me with any questions you might have throughout your pregnancy. This book will be published in over 10 languages simultaneously, and I may receive a fair number of questions – so if you can, try to keep your questions within the scope of this project.

In closing this book, I'd like to wish you the best for the journey of your pregnancy.[26] I have two kids myself, and the powerful joy, energy and happiness of the event of their births is something I carry with me every day.

At that time, I didn't have a full grasp on the elements that make up the foundation of this book. As a child, though, I lost my beloved grandmother when she fell into a diabetic coma and passed away a few hours later. I've distrusted sugar ever since, and I consume it in only very moderate amounts. My wife feels the same.

So, without knowing the epigenetic explanation under-lying it, my wife's diet during her pregnancies was fairly close to what I have recommended in this book. What's more, back then (my eldest child was born thirty-three years ago), industrial food hadn't reached the intense degree of transformation of today's foods. My children were born with a normal weight, and they have no problem controlling their weight today.

---

[26] For any information, email me at: p.dukan60@gmail.com

My deep love for my family inspires me to protect them, which is why I mention them here – and I know that the same motivation is guiding you. The plan in this book takes that motivation a step further: it aims to make your pregnancy, and every pregnancy, a healthy one. Through this plan, we share a common goal. Thank you for joining me. I'll support you every step of the way.

References and
Further Reading

1. World Health Organization (WHO), 'Obesity and Diabetes', Fact Sheet #311, Epidemiological Survey, 2009

2. *Obesity Reviews*, 2016 from the International Association for the Study of Obesity (IASO)

3. www.ligue-cancer.net/article/6397_leschiffres-cles-des-cancers

4. Anderson, R.J., Freedland, K.E., Clouse R.E. and Lustman, P.J., *The Prevalence of Comorbid Depression in Adults with Diabetes, Diabet. Med.*, Nov. 23 2006, 23

5. Luppino, F.S., det Wit, L.M., et al, 'Overweight, obesity and depression: a systematic review and meta-analysis of longitudinal studies', *Arch. Gen. Psychiatry*, March 2010, 67 (3)

6. www.databank.banquemondiale.org/data/ reports www.oecd.org/fr/env/indicateurs-modelisation-perspectives/49884240.pdf

7. Sacks, F.M., Bray, G.A., Carey, V.J. et al., 'Comparison of weight-loss diets with different compositions of fat, protein and carbohydrates', The New England Journal of Medicine, 2009, 360 (9)

8. www.lanutrition.fr

9. www.youtube.com/watch?v=dBnniua6

10. IASO, 27 May 2014 (www.oecd.org/health/obesity-update)

11. Reece, A. Leguizamón, G. Wiznitzer, A. 'Gestational diabetes: the need for a common ground', Lancet, 2009; 73

12. Guillaume, Jean, *Ils ont domestique plantes et animaux. Prelude a la civilisation*, (translation) Quae Editions, 2011

13. *Lancet*, 5 October 2013, vol. 382, No. 9899

14. La Recherche, April 2012, 463

15. Rosnay, Joel de, 'La grande revolution de la biologie de ces cinq dernieres annees – pas dix, vint, trente: cinq dernieres annees'

16. Miller, Jennie Brand, Marsh, Kate and Moses, Robert, *The Bump to Baby Low GI Eating Plan*, Hachette Australia, 2012

17. *La Recherche*, April 2012, *op cit*

18. Charles, M.A., L'unite mixte Ined-Inserm-EFS

19. 'Medicine and Research', Seminar 12 of the IPSEN Foundation, Endocrinology Series

20. University of Southampton, 'New link between mother's pregnancy diet and offspring's chances of obesity' study, 2011

21. Hanson, M., Gluckman, P., 'Developmental origins of non-communicable disease: Population and public health implications', *American Journal of Clinical Nutrition*, 2011, 94

REFERENCES

22. 'Medicine and Research', Seminar 12 of the IPSEN Foundation, Endocrinology Series

23. www.thousanddays.org

24. Lenoir, M., Serre, F. and Ahmed, S.H., 'Intense sweetness surpasses cocaine reward', *PLoS One*, August 2007, 1; 2(8). Universite Bordeaux, CNRS, UMR 5227.

25. *Le Monde: Science and Technology*, 28 April 2012

Further Reading

1. McGrath, J. Solter, D. 'Completion of embryogenesis requires both the maternal and paternal genomes'. *Cell*, 1984; 37: 179–83.

2. Surani, M.A. Barton, S. Norris, M. 'Development of reconstituted mouse eggs suggests imprinting of the genome during gametogenesis'. *Nature*, 1984; 308: 548–50.

3. Cattanach, B.M. Kirk, M. 'Differential activity of maternally and paternally derived chromosome regions in mice'. *Nature*, 1985; 315: 496–8.

4. Cattanach, B.M. Beechey, C.V. Peters, J. 'Interactions between imprinting effects in the mouse'. *Genetics*, 2004; 168: 397–413.

5. DeChiara, T.M. Efstratiadis, A. Robertson, E.J. 'A growth deficiency phenotype in heterozygous mice carrying an insulin-like growth factor II gene disrupted by gene targeting'. *Nature*, 1990; 345: 78–80. *Revues Synthèse* 395 TIRÉS À PART L. Dandolo.

6. Barlow, D.P. Stöger, R. Hermann, B.G. et al. 'The mouse insulin-like growth factor type 2 receptor is imprinted and closely linked to the Tme locus'. *Nature*, 1991; 349: 84–7.

7. Li, E. Bestor, T.H. Jaenisch R. 'Targeted mutation of the

DNA methyltransferase gene results in embryonic lethality'. *Cell*, 1992; 69: 915–26.

8. Hata, K. Okano, M. Lei, H. Li, E, 'Dnmt3L cooperates with the Dnmt3 family of de novo DNA methyltransferases to establish maternal imprints in mice'. *Development*, 2002; 129: 1983–93.

9. Bourc'his, D. Xu, G.L. Lin, C.S. et al. 'Dnmt3L and the establishment of maternal genomic imprints'. *Science*, 2001; 294: 2536–9.

10. Li, E. 'Chromatin modification and epigenetic reprogramming in mammalian development'. *Nat Rev Genet*, 2002; 3: 662–73.

11. Mager, J. Montgomery, N.D. de Villena, F.P. Magnuson, T. 'Genome imprinting regulated by the mouse Polycomb group protein Eed'. *Nat Genet*, 2003; 33: 502–7.

12. Umlauf, D. Goto, Y. Cao, R. et al. 'Imprinting along the Kcnq1 domain on mouse chromosome 7 involves repressive histone methylation and recruitment of Polycomb group complexes'. *Nat Genet*, 2004; 36: 1296–300.

13. Lewis, A. Mitsuya K. Umlauf D. et al. 'Imprinting on distal chromosome 7 in the placenta involves repressive histone methylation independent of DNA methylation'. *Nat Genet*, 2004; 36: 1291–5.

14. Reik, W. Dean, W. Walter, J. Epigenetic reprogramming in mammalian development'. *Science*, 2001; 293: 1089–93.

15. Lucifero, D. Mann, M.R. Bartolomei, M.S. Trasler, J.M. 'Gene-specific timing and epigenetic memory in oocyte imprinting'. *Hum Mol Genet*, 2004; 13: 839–49.

16. Obata, Y. Kaneko-Ishino, T. Koide, T. et al. 'Disruption of

primary imprinting during oocyte growth leads to the modified expression of imprinted genes during embryogenesis'. *Development*, 1998; 125: 1553–60.

17. Kono, T. Obata, Y. Wu, Q. et al. 'Birth of parthenogenetic mice that can develop to adulthood'. *Nature*, 2004; 428: 860–4.

18. Lopes, S. Lewis, A. Hajkova, P. et al. 'Epigenetic modifications in an imprinting cluster are controlled by a hierarchy of DMRs suggesting long-range chromatin interactions'. *Hum Mol Genet*, 2003; 12: 295–305.

19. Hark, A.T. Schoenherr, C.J. Katz, D.J. et al. 'CTCF mediates methylation-sensitive enhancer-blocking activity at the H19/Igf2 locus'. *Nature*, 2000; 405: 486–9.

20. Lee, M.P. DeBaun, M.R. Mitsuya, K. et al. 'Loss of imprinting of a paternally expressed transcript, with antisense orientation to KVLQT1, occurs frequently in BeckwithWiedemann syndrome and is independent of insulin-like growth factor II imprinting'. *Proc Natl Acad Sci USA*, 1999; 96: 5203–8.

21. Wutz, A. Smrzka, O.W. Schweifer, N. et al. 'Imprinted expression of the Igf2r gene depends on an intronic CpG island' *Nature*, 1997; 389: 745–9.

22. Sleutels, F. Zwart, R. Barlow, D.P. 'The non-coding Air RNA is required for silencing autosomal imprinted genes'. *Nature*, 2002; 415 : 810–13.

23. Rougeulle, C. Cardoso, C. Fontes, M. et al. 'An imprinted antisense RNA overlaps UBE3A and a second maternally expressed transcript'. *Nat Genet*, 1998; 19: 15–16.

24. Landers, M. Bancescu, D.L. Le Meur, E. et al. 'Regulation of the large (approximately 1000 kb) imprinted murine Ube3a

antisense transcript by alternative exons upstream of Snurf/ Snrpn'. *Nucleic Acids Res*, 2004; 32: 3480–92.

25. Rougeulle, C. Heard, E. 'Antisense RNA in imprinting: spreading silence through Air'. *Trends Genet*, 2002; 18: 434–7.

26. Thakur, N. Tiwari, V.K. Thomassin, H. et al. 'An antisense RNA regulates the bidirectional silencing property of the Kcnq1 imprinting control region'. *Mol Cell Biol*, 2004; 24: 7855–62.

27. Verona, R.I. Mann, M.R. Bartolomei, M.S. 'Genomic imprinting: intricacies of epigenetic regulation in clusters'. *Annu Rev Cell Dev Biol*, 2003; 19: 237–59.

28. Drewell, R.A. Brenton, J.D. Ainscough, J.F. et al. 'Deletion of a silencer element disrupts H19 imprinting independently of a DNA methylation epigenetic switch'. *Development*, 2000; 127: 3419–28.

29. Gosden, R. Trasler, J. Lucifero, D. Faddy, M. 'Rare congenital disorders', imprint.

General Reading

May 2016 study into the Impact of Maternal Glucose and Gestational Weight Gain on Child Obesity over the First Decade of Life in Normal Birth Weight Infant: Hillier, T.A., Pedula, K.L., Vesco, K.K. et al. Matern Child Health J (2016) 20: 1559. doi:10.1007/s10995-016-1955-7

www.sciencedaily.com/releases/2016/05/160506095656

For more information, and to monitor your pregnancy nutrition (as explained on page 239), visit www.baby6months.com Dr Pierre Dukan's free-to-use website, with food lists and an online journal to monitor all your nutritional needs through pregnancy.